Shepherds of Destiny II

EVIL ACROSS TIME

KIEL BARNEKOV

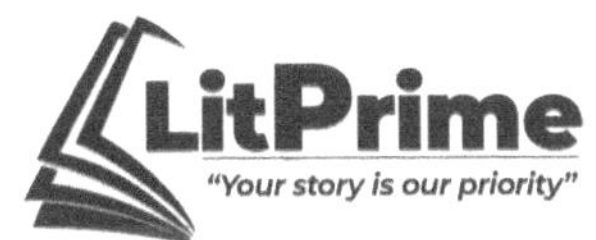

LitPrime Solutions
21250 Hawthorne Blvd
Suite 500, Torrance, CA 90503
www.litprime.com
Phone: 1-800-981-9893

Published by LitPrime Solutions   04/28/2023

ISBN: 979-8-88703-128-6(sc)
ISBN: 979-8-88703-242-9(hc)
ISBN: 979-8-88703-129-3(e)

Library of Congress Control Number: 2022923711

Contents

Prologue

In the late 2030s, a cyborg or synthetic body had been developed by a Defense Advanced Research Projects Agency (DARPA) team led by Dr. Ansley Barnett that fully resembled the human body. To the untrained eye, the cyborg body was indistinguishable from a human body. The cyborg was controlled by a human mind, downloaded to the electronic brain from a patient irreversibly incapacitated by a disease or accident. The cyborg could eat and drink when desired in order to better blend with the human population. Food was 'digested' by the synthetic body by reducing anything ingested to a gas and cleansed of any odor before excretion. Its senses mirrored the senses of a human. It did not require sleep, although it periodically needed to rest the human mind it was hosting and recharge its advanced battery array, which was located where the kidneys are on a human body. It could enjoy having sex.

Kristian Barnett, a billionaire through inheritance of his parents' estate, and CEO and Chairman of the Board of Barnett Industries which developed, manufactured and implemented advanced transportation systems globally, fell ill at thirty-three with amyotrophic lateral sclerosis (ALS), also known as Lou Gehrig's Disease.

Dr. Savannah Richards, Neurosurgeon and Research Scientist at the Stanford Neuroscience Health Center was developing a means to preserve the brain of a patient whose body had been irrecoverably destroyed but whose brain was unharmed. Concurrently, Dr. Ansley Barnett, wife of Kristian Barnett, was leading the development of a cyborg body indistinguishable from a human body for DARPA.

Soon after Kristian's brain was removed and placed in stasis, he was approached by The Guardian. The Guardian was a spiritual being who watched for timelines that were going astray and threatening the existence of humanity. The Guardian needed Kristian's mind, untethered from his corporeal body, to control the actions of key individuals. While in his current spiritual state, Kristian could travel to any period in the past or future with The Guardian to affect changes to a timeline gone astray.

With Kristian in tow, The Guardian traveled back in time to the U.S. Civil War, where the timeline in which the Union won the war was in jeopardy. With Kristian's mind in brief control of one key individual, the catastrophe was averted, and history continued its pre-destined course.

Aaron Adams, also suffering from advanced ALS, was approved as a candidate for the brain extraction procedure. But unlike Kristian, prior to the procedure his mind would be scanned and stored for download to a cyborg body. The download was a complete success and Aaron was introduced back into society under a new identity. Aaron was also approached by The Guardian, as his mind was also separated from his corporeal body. His assignment from The Guardian resulted in the timeline being maintained in which the Allies won World War II and defeated the Axis Alliance of Germany, Italy and Japan.

Commander Erik Richards, captain of the Mars spaceship USS Elon Musk, was returning to Earth from Mars when the ship experienced a catastrophic hull breach that led to the deaths of four of her crew and inflicted extensive wounds on Erik. The prognosis for Erik was that he would not recover beyond a quadriplegic state. It was then approved for Erik to receive a synthetic cyborg body.

A crewmember with whom Erik was developing a relationship, Technical Specialist Arya Anderson, was killed. Nearly a year after the accident aboard the Musk, after Erik had completed his transition to a synthetic body, Erik traveled to Arya's home in Norway to meet with her grieving parents and siblings. While there, Erik and Arya's sister, Ksenia, fell in love and their relationship continues in this book.

Kristian Barnett and Aaron Adams, under the guidance of The Guardian, traveled forward to the year 2052. The CEO of Find Corporation and two multi-billion-dollar telecommunication moguls had developed a new smartphone supporting an advanced communications technology. This technology enabled the ability to control a user's thoughts and actions without the knowledge or consent of the user. The new smartphone and communications technology were promoted to the military as a means of controlling the actions of an enemy. The intent of the billionaire cabal was to use the technology to establish a dystopian world in which the billionaire elites and their ruling class government puppets would live in opulence while the masses were enslaved to serve their masters.

The demonstration of the technology to senior government officials, including the Secretary of Defense, was a failure due to the intervention of Kristian and Aaron taking brief control of the test subjects' and SecDef's minds. Although successfully stalled, the CEO of Find vowed to correct the cause of the failure and offered to fund whatever amount was necessary.

Upon their return from the future, Kristian questioned The Guardian whether the effort to develop the mind control technology could be accomplished prior to 2052. The Guardian agreed it was possible, but that it would be exceedingly difficult, even dangerous, to alter a timeline. Kristian and Aaron then worked with Senator Richards, Erik's and Savannah's uncle, and DARPA to gain participation in the project to develop the technology.

Chapter One

"Aaron, can you come up to my office?" said Kristian. "I want to discuss your upcoming trip to meet with the Find Corporation team working on the mind control project."

"Be right up," said Aaron, sitting at his desk in the Barnett Center for Neurologic Restoration and appearing to speak to no one. His smartwatch picked up his voice and transmitted his response to Kristian. He then rose to take the elevator down to the lower level of the building and catch the Transporter, essentially a vacuum tube between Barnett Center and the Barnett mansion that worked virtually like the vacuum tube in a bank drive-up window. After entering the Transporter car, Aaron found himself in the lower lobby of the mansion in five seconds, although it was three-fourths of a mile from the Center. He experienced no effects from the sudden, extreme acceleration and speed. Barnett Industry Transporter systems were installed in several cities in the United States and internationally, replacing old, slow subways in many of them.

A few minutes later, in Kristian's elaborate office in the Barnett mansion, Aaron took a seat across from Kristian, who was sitting behind an ornate desk that had originally belonged to Kristian's father. The desk was carved from rare Cuban mahogany and drew one's attention immediately upon entering the room. Behind the desk was a matching credenza and hutch. The hutch comprised an open area that contained a painting of the Barnett mansion, bordered by glass-door cabinets that held mementos accumulated mostly by Kristian's father during his career as founder and head of Barnett Industries.

"Good morning, Aaron. I just got off the phone with Jonathon Brahe. He mentioned that the teams from Cyclone Networks and Networks Affiliated had received their top-secret clearance and will meet next week at Find headquarters. You should plan on attending in person. I would go as well, but I'm not ready to allow a room full of strangers to see me in person. I am planning on attending via holoconference."

"I've continued my research into the likely means of delivering electromagnetic energy to the human brain," said Aaron. "There were several attempts made by several governments at disrupting the brain using microwaves. In late 2016 and early 2017 there were reports of personnel assigned to the American embassy in Cuba suffering symptoms of electromagnetic radiation sickness. The medical team that studied the U.S. diplomats in Cuba ascribed the symptoms to 'an unknown energy source' that was highly directional. Some personnel, it noted, had covered their ears and heads but experienced no sound reduction. The team said the diplomats appeared to have developed signs of concussion without having received any blows to the head."

"It is common knowledge that microwaves are ubiquitous in modern life. The short radio waves power radars, cook foods, relay messages, and link cellphones to antenna towers. Barnett Industries' proprietary cellular technology employs microwaves to generate commands to networked city transportation grids and to vehicles of all types for traffic control," said Kristian. "So microwaves can deliver information in a manner that disrupts human thought."

"Exactly. One means of delivering directed microwaves involves the use of a simple telecommunications dish that can be mobile. And what we saw when we went forward in time to 2052 was evidently a perfected state of microwave technology delivery being used to alter the reality of the human target."

"Has there been any efforts at legislation rendering the use of electromagnetic technology to affect the human mind illegal?" asked Kristian.

"There was a bill introduced in the U.S. House of Representatives back in 2001 that included a ban on the use of electromagnetic radiation aimed at individuals, among several other uses of technology. The bill never made it to the House Floor for a vote. There was also a Senate hearing chaired by Senator Marco Rubio in 2017 to investigate the situation experienced by the U.S. diplomats in Cuba, which resulted in no action being taken."

"So, what we saw in our trip forward to 2052 was a device that appeared to be a smartphone used to deliver messages to a human subject that changed or altered the subject's reality. The message was delivered via a cellular network in a manner not dissimilar in concept to the way Barnett Industries delivers instructions to various transportation systems and vehicles. Of course, delivering a message that can alter the reality of a biological being is an order of magnitude more complex than delivering messages to software and hardware," said Kristian.

"Indeed, what is needed for Find to achieve their goal will require the transmission of instructions encapsulated in just the right frequency and strength of microwave energy. The delivery device—the smartphone—necessary to achieve this will be the key to Find's success. If the microwave energy is too strong, it could cause injury to the user. If it is too weak, the data may not be correctly delivered. Either way, the intent of the message is lost and is therefore unsuccessful."

"Regarding the meeting with the Find team, I suggest we attend, intending to be primarily an observer. Let's try to determine Find's strategy for developing their course of action along with their telecommunications partners. As the successor to much of the old Google empire after the court-mandated split up in the late 2020s, Find is still manufacturing cellular devices using the Android operating system. So, Find will be the one to design and develop the signal delivery device as a smartphone we saw used in 2052," said Kristian. "I'll have KB (Kristian's personal digital assistant) make your travel arrangements and setup the holoconference for me."

Aaron nodded and got up to leave Kristian's office when Kristian said, "By the way, how are things going between Savannah and you? Are you two still a 'thing'?"

"Going great. We've had several dates and are planning a weekend together soon," replied Aaron. "Savannah is an extremely smart, talented, and beautiful woman. Every time I am with her, I see myself getting fonder of her. I hope she's thinking the same way about me."

"I certainly agree with you, Aaron. Savannah is quite a girl. You'd be extremely hard pressed to find a better partner."

Chapter Two

L t. Scarlett Bross, the naval aviator who had lost her left arm and leg in the accident aboard the USS Trump, had been moved to the Barnett Center for Neurological Restoration shortly after her initial interview with Drs. Ansley Barnett and Savannah Richards at the Veterans Administration hospital in San Diego. Lt. Bross had been briefed on the procedure needed to restore full body functions. Her brain would be scanned, and her mind uploaded to a massive database where it could then be downloaded into the electronic brain in a synthetic body — a cyborg. To the untrained eye, she would be indistinguishable from her human body. Her synthetic body would not age naturally but could be altered to simulate aging if she desired. The synthetic body could emulate all human functions, including those of all her senses. She could enjoy eating and having sex. Today, Drs. Barnett and Richards would show her the synthetic body that her mind would occupy indefinitely.

Drs. Barnett and Richards appeared at her door, dressed in their traditional white medical coats. "Scarlett, are you ready to see your future?" asked Ansley Barnett.

"I... I think so," replied Scarlett.

"Good, we'll take the elevator down to the lower level, where lab operations are located. We think you'll be pleasantly surprised at what you are about to see," said Ansley.

Exiting the elevator, they turned right and proceeded through a set of stainless-steel double doors to the cyborg lab. On a table resembling an operating table, the shape of a body covered head-to-toe by a sheet could be seen. The table was bordered by several workstations, each with computer screens producing data on the state of the systems supporting the cyborg.

Ansley walked in front of Scarlett's wheelchair and stood between Scarlett and the body on the metal operating table. "Are you ready, Scarlett? I hope this won't be too great a shock for you."

"Yes, I'm ready," said Scarlett, unconsciously holding her breath.

Ansley then removed the sheet, exposing the synthetic body. The synthetic was identical in appearance to Scarlett except that it was whole, with all four limbs and no visible scars from the accident aboard the USS Donald Trump where Scarlett's F-35 missed the deck and bounced into the South China Sea during nighttime pitching deck exercises. Immediately startled, Scarlett inhaled sharply as she saw the synthetic body for the first time. "That is… incredible," she stammered. "That… she… I need a moment."

"We understand," said Savannah. "Remember, the transition to this synthetic body will not only erase your wounds completely, but it will also give you a much stronger body that could last indefinitely. No aging, no disease, no hunger or thirst, no pain."

Scarlett was speechless for what seemed like minutes but was only several seconds. "This is the most incredible thing I've ever seen," she said as she broke down in tears. "I did not know science had advanced this far. But I do have many questions."

"We expected you would," said Savannah. "Why don't we go up to my office where we can provide you with more information and answer your questions. I believe there will be someone whom you've not previously met waiting for us."

As Savannah led the three into her office, she was immediately grabbed and hugged by a man in a tan Navy uniform. "Hey, sis, great to see you!" said Commander Erik Richards.

"Wonderful seeing you, Erik!" said Savannah. "I'd like you to meet someone," as she stepped aside from the front of Scarlett's wheelchair. "This is Scarlett Bross, Lt. Scarlett Bross, naval aviator."

"Nice to finally meet you, Lieutenant," said Erik. "I've heard a lot about you. Sorry about your accident. Those pitching deck landings are terrifying."

"Sorry, I'm not able to stand, sir," said Scarlett. "Good to meet you, too. I've heard a lot about you and your accident, as well as your… transition."

"Please call me Erik. Savannah and Ansley asked me to come out here and give you some insight into what is about to happen to you and answer questions you may have. I can say that my entire experience can only be described as miraculous. I understand you just saw the future you. Any thoughts?"

"I guess I'm still overwhelmed even though I had seen pictures of the… synthetic body, as well as video of you during your recovery period. The videos were quite impressive."

"Ansley and I will leave you two to get acquainted," said Savannah. "Let's meet in the cafeteria at 1:00 PM for lunch."

"What can I tell you about my experience and what to expect," said Erik. "May I call you Scarlett?"

"Of course. Start with what you felt as soon as you awoke from the download," said Scarlett. "Did you feel any pain or unusual sensation?"

"I recall that when I first opened my eyes and saw Ansley looking down at me so intensely, I thought I might be dead. For what seemed like minutes, I could not move. I could not even blink my eyes or make any expression to let anyone know I was… there. Then I could see my sister and I somehow came to life. Savannah asked me if I knew where I was and I replied, 'On Mars.' She got this terribly concerned look on her face when I smiled at her. She immediately hit my shoulder, which I actually felt and scolded me for joking around at such a serious time."

"Oh my God, you were joking as you were waking up in your synthetic body?" laughed Scarlett. "I think I would've pulled the plug on you right there! Did you have any concerns or hesitation with the procedure? I know I have some concerns."

"Well, the idea of completely abandoning my corporeal body was scary. But when I considered I would probably be a physical vegetable for the rest of my life, I knew that for me it was my only option. But I believe I was in a worse place than you are physically. About the only thing I could do on my own was breathe. And that only after a couple of months on a respirator. You at least have some mobility and control of your right arm and leg. What you need to decide is are you willing to live the rest of your life in half of a body. Going from the flight deck of an F-35 to a wheelchair is an almost unimaginable situation. The best you could probably hope for is an assignment flying drones, like flying a video game."

Scarlett just sat and stared out the window of Savannah's office for several minutes. She then turned to Erik, with tears running down her cheeks, and said, "Looking at you and seeing how you have recovered and moved on with your career, doing what you love, gives me hope I can do the same. Nothing would make me happier than climbing into an F-35 and catapulting off the deck with my hair on fire. But I still seem to have reservations. Have you had a relationship since recovering? I'm concerned that I won't be looked at as a… woman, but as a robot."

"Now that you mention it, yes, I am currently in a relationship with a beautiful woman. Her name is Ksenia. She is the sister of Arya Anderson, who died in the accident aboard the Musk. We met when I went to Norway to meet Arya's family and share their grief over the loss of their daughter. Ksenia is a Second Mate on a Viking Cruise Lines ship and currently on a cruise in the Med. She will be on leave soon, and we plan to spend as much time together as possible."

"What does Ksenia think about your… condition?" asked Scarlett.

"Full disclosure. Ksenia does not know about my condition. This is partially because I am a state secret. I am strictly prohibited from disclosing my condition to anyone not approved by SecDef and DARPA. You will be under the same non-disclosure rules indefinitely. But I do plan to tell Ksenia at the appropriate time, after securing permission from the proper authorities."

"So, you and Ksenia have made love and she couldn't tell you are… synthetic?"

"My Scarlett, you are direct! I should've seen that coming, especially from a fellow aviator," laughed Erik. "The answer is yes to both questions."

"Well, that's encouraging, I guess. You can get that close to someone, and they cannot tell you're not… corporeal."

"Is there someone special in your life that is spawning these emotions in you?" asked Erik.

"Not really. I mean, there is a pilot that I met on our last cruise. We seemed to hit it off pretty well. He came to see me in San Diego at the VA hospital a couple of times. But it's nothing serious, at least not yet."

"What other concerns do you have regarding your transition?"

"Will I be able to have children?" said Scarlett.

"Would you still be able to have children in your human body?"

Scarlett hesitated, looked down, and then said, "No, my uterus was damaged in the accident."

"Then I suggest you address that question to Ansley, but it doesn't sound like having children should be an issue with completing your transition."

"What about maintaining your synthetic body, Erik? Do you have to get regular maintenance, oil changes, or tune-ups?" asked Scarlett.

"I must visit the Center every six months and go through a battery of tests on all my body systems. I also must sit down with the Center's psychiatrist, Dr. Samuel McKensey, so he can assure Ansley that I will not turn into a transformer."

"It is getting close to 1300. Let's go down to the cafeteria to meet Ansley and Savannah," said Erik.

Erik pushed Scarlett's wheelchair down the hall to the elevator, where the two descended to the first-floor company cafeteria. As they entered the cafeteria, they ran into Aaron Adams.

"Erik? Hello! Pleasure to see you," said Aaron.

"Hey Aaron, how have you been?"

"Fantastic. Are you two having lunch?"

"Yes, we're meeting Savannah and Ansley. Why don't you join us? By the way, this is Scarlett Bross, a fellow naval aviator."

"Pleased to meet you, Scarlett," said Aaron. "I will join you. I was going to see if I could run into Savannah, anyway."

Just then, Savannah and Ansley appeared at the entrance to the cafeteria. "Hey, guys, anybody feel like lunch today?" said Ansley.

They all entered the cafeteria buffet, and either ordered from the grill or grabbed a pre-made salad. The ladies selected a variety of salads, declining the included serving of bread and butter, while the cyborgs ordered cheeseburgers and fries from the grill. They then found a round table that accommodated the group comfortably.

"Still no sympathy for us girls trying to maintain our figures, I see," said Ansley. "Scarlett, you'll see these cyborgs chow down on all the fat and carbs they want while we eat bunny food. At least you can look forward to eating whatever you want after your transition."

"When will you be transitioning, Scarlett?" asked Aaron.

"I'll have to refer that question to Ansley, but I think it is to be scheduled soon."

"We have everything ready and are just running some final tests on the network to make sure everything is optimal for the download of Scarlett to the synthetic body," said Ansley. "I believe we'll be a go by early next week."

Chapter Three

It is October 7, 2042. Aaron Adams (aka Phillip Preston) has arrived in the lobby of Find Corporation's corporate headquarters in Mountain View, California. "Good morning, Mr. Preston, please look into the scanner there on the desk," said a voice attached to the holographic image of an attractive young woman projected behind the reception desk. His retina was scanned, and the file embedded in a visitor's identification badge. "Thank you, Mr. Preston. Mr. Brahe's assistant will be down to meet you momentarily. You can wait by the fountain behind you." The holographic image disappeared.

Aaron then heard the click of heels approaching him from behind. Turning he heard, "Good morning, Mr. Preston. My name is Jillian, and I will show you up to the executive offices and conference room for your meeting with Mr. Brahe. Please follow me."

"Good morning, Jillian. This building is quite impressive," said Aaron, thinking that Jillian was quite attractive. They stepped into an elevator where Jillian looked into a scanner and said, "twelfth floor." When they arrived, Aaron followed Jillian to a large conference room. Aaron noticed that there were no windows in the room. But Jillian touched a button on the wall near the double doors and the opposite wall dissolved into a bank of floor-to-ceiling windows with a view overlooking the Find Corporation campus twelve stories below.

"Mr. Brahe will be with you in a few moments," said Jillian, who turned and exited the conference room.

Aaron was looking out over the Find campus when Jonathon Brahe entered the conference room. "Good morning, Phillip. I hope you had a pleasant trip up from Bel-Air. The people from Cyclone and Networks Affiliated will be here shortly. Can I get you a cup of coffee or some water or fruit juice?"

"No thanks. I'm good for now. Can we setup the holoconference for Kristian to attend?"

"Certainly," said Jonathon. He then waved his hand in front of a spot outlined on the wall to his left and an area around one chair at the table became enshrouded in a gray rectangular box. "Here is the URL for Kristian to access when he is ready. He will appear in the chair outlined at the table."

Jonathon Brahe began the meeting by introducing the team members. "From Cyclone Networks we have Jennifer Briton and Jeremy Stringer. Jennifer is the head of Cyclone's advanced wireless division. Jeremy is Cyclone's chief engineer. From Networks Affiliated, Jason Bannon, senior vice president of networks and Barbara Braden, head of research and development. From Barnett Industries, Kristian Barnett, CEO, and Phillip Preston, senior vice president of research and development. Finally, besides myself from Find, are Jane True and James Handley. Jane heads up R&D and James oversees software development."

"Now, I should remind everyone that we are all under strict non-disclosure agreements with the federal government. Violation of those agreements comes with severe penalties, including jail time. Please keep that in mind when you deal with the media or other third parties. I will now ask Jane to present the latest equipment that may provide the delivery vehicle for our mind-altering technology. Jane."

Jane opened a box placed in front of her seat at the table. The black box measured approximately nine by nine inches. She took a device that was approximately eight inches by four inches in her hand and held it up. It appeared to be an ordinary, clear-glass oval smartphone.

"Ladies and gentlemen, this device may appear to be a harmless smartphone like those that each of you currently carry. And it provides all the functions and apps your smartphones offer. However, there is a second CPU and memory running internal to this device that, with the proper advanced software, can produce commands for transmission to the user. James, would you like to speak to the envisioned capabilities of the software for this device?"

"Thanks, Jane. Good morning ladies and gentlemen. Jane mentioned the device can produce commands for delivery to the user, or target, of the device. What we envision for this device is a library of commands that could potentially control what a user is perceiving around them that could cause a desired decision by the user. An operator in a remote location would generate a signal to the device via a cellular network or satellite link that would tell the device which command, or series of commands to generate to the target. The command would then be delivered to the user via a tiny microwave generator incorporated into the smartphone. A simple execution might be to change the target's perception of the weather. On a bright sunny day, an operator sends a command. The smartphone knows the actual weather at its location, so it then knows what weather conditions to include in the command to the target. The smartphone then generates the description of the altered weather, let's say rainy, windy conditions via a microwave signal sent directly into the brain of the target. Upon calling the target using the smartphone, one asks the target what the weather is currently. The target, looking out a nearby window, sees that it is raining and windy."

"Impressive," said Kristian Barnett. "But what technology is being used to plant subliminal suggestions into the brain of the target that will actually result in changing his perception of what he/she is looking at?"

"Thank you, Kristian, for asking that important question," said Jonathan Brahe. "In the late 2010s and early 2020s, a technology that became known as BCI, Brain-Computer Interface, was in early development. BCI was to provide a means for the mind, using the brain of its host, to issue outbound commands to robotic and semi-robotic instruments. They embedded sensors in the brain at strategic locations that would react to thoughts by the host and generate commands. Ultra-thin wires were used to transmit the signals from the neurons to a machine. The technology was mostly conceptual but involved experimentation on rats. As the technology developed through the 2020s into the 2030s, the wired portion of the technology was replaced with wireless technology. The neuro-sensors still had to be surgically implanted in the brain, but the wires to the machinery were eliminated. Neurons can be stimulated non-invasively by delivering pulsed magnetic fields through the skull (TMS), by applying DC or AC current into the brain through electrodes on the scalp, and by beaming ultrasound into neural tissue. None of these currently have the microscopic precision that an implanted electrode has to stimulate a single neuron, but they do influence neural circuit function, and they don't require surgery. BCI technology is now used for the control of artificial limbs, where the target can control an artificial limb by simply using thought. Today, research is continuing to explore the science of introducing commands into the human brain."

"So, if I understand correctly, the challenge is to stimulate a specific neuron or neurons to elicit a specific reaction by the target without the target's knowledge or awareness. I believe that the Barnett Center for Neurological Restoration may contribute to the development of this technology," said Kristian. "Dr. Savannah Richards is one of a handful of preeminent scientists in neurology. You may have heard her name associated with the cure for Alzheimer's disease in the late 2020s. Dr. Richards is behind the development of a cure for ALS, which is how I can take part in this meeting today. I recommend she be added to the team as soon as possible." Kristian glanced at Aaron and could see that Aaron understood why Kristian offered to enlist Savannah on the project. She would provide a fantastic opportunity to not only develop the medical technology to generate commands subliminally to targets, but to develop the virus necessary to kill the technology.

"I am familiar with Dr. Richards' work, Kristian," said Jonathon. "From what I know, I agree she would be a valuable asset to this team. Will you get with our DARPA project manager, Inger Beck, and coordinate getting the clearance for Dr. Richards?"

"Of course."

Chapter Four

"Scarlett, from your perspective, the procedure for transitioning you to your synthetic body is rather simple. We will start by giving you a sedative to relax you. Shortly afterward, we will administer the anesthesia that will render you unconscious. The next thing you will experience will be awakening in your new body. At first, you will probably experience disorientation and confusion. That will pass as you regain consciousness. From there, we will begin testing the ability of your mind to control the synthetic body. You will be asked to perform actions like wiggling your toes, moving arms and legs, and responding to stimulation of your senses. Do you have questions?" said Ansley.

"What will be done with my… human body?" asked Scarlett.

"We will keep it comatose for the period we deem necessary to ensure that your synthetic body is functioning properly," said Ansley.

"And after that is determined?" said Scarlett.

"We will discuss the disposition of your human body with you. Any action taken will be done with your full knowledge and approval."

"What did the other cyborgs–Kristian, Aaron, and Erik–do with their human bodies?"

"I am not at liberty to disclose that information, but you may ask them that question yourself. Are you ready to proceed with the transition?"

"Yes, I am ready."

"All systems are green to go with the download," said OR technician Janice.

"Start download," said Ansley.

Ninety-six seconds later Janice said, "Download complete."

"Start data distribution," said Ansley. The electronic brain of the cyborg began populating the scanned data from Scarlett's mind in the targeted areas of its brain.

"Data distribution complete," said Janice, after thirty-three minutes, forty seconds. "Download process complete."

Ansley moved closer to the synthetic body created in the image of Scarlett Bross laying on the metal table. She shined the light from a small LED flashlight on the cyborg's closed eyes. The eyes opened, and the dilated pupils contracted, which was an autonomous reaction by the cyborg which showed brain function was active.

"Scarlett, can you hear me?" said Ansley. "Scarlett, are you with us?"

Nothing moved on the cyborg's face. No sign of recognition or reaction to Ansley's voice could be seen.

"Scarlett!" said Ansley, her voice increasing in volume.

The cyborg's eyes fluttered and focused on the sound of Ansley's voice.

"Scarlett, blink once if you can hear my voice."

The cyborg blinked slowly.

"Scarlett, can you speak?"

Scarlett opened her mouth slightly and emitted a sound like that of a deep sigh.

"She is definitely understanding you," said Savannah to Ansley.

"Scarlett, how do you feel? Are you in any discomfort?"

Scarlett appeared to be straining and then said, "Good," through a sound resembling compressed gas escaping from a tank.

"Scarlett, we are going to test your reaction to external stimuli. We will start by testing your sense of feel with this needle. Please indicate whether you feel the needle by saying 'yes'." Ansley then touched the needle to Scarlett's right arm from her shoulder to her palm. Scarlett said, "yes" to each prick of the needle. Ansley then performed similar tests on Scarlett's right leg from hip to heel, with the same result.

"Scarlett, I am going to perform the same tests on your left arm and leg." Ansley stuck the needle in Scarlett's right shoulder. Scarlett responded positively. But as Ansley began moving the point of the needle down Scarlett's left arm towards her wrist, Scarlett stopped responding. It was apparent that Scarlett could not feel the needle.

"Scarlett, I have pressed the needle into your arm several times," said Ansley. "Did you feel it?"

"No," replied Scarlett.

"That's OK, we will continue to test over the next several days. With Erik, testing showed that he could not feel his legs at first. It was our conclusion that since he had been paralyzed for several months, his mind had temporarily lost its ability to receive sensations from the paralyzed limbs. This condition may be what we are seeing with your limbs that were amputated. It will most likely resolve in a short time. I will test your left leg now."

The same condition was reflected testing Scarlett's left leg. "Scarlett, please continue to move your left fingers and toes. You will need to concentrate. Try to visualize your fingers and toes moving in your mind."

Several minutes passed and there was no apparent movement of Scarlett's fingers or toes. "OK, let's proceed with testing Scarlett's basic mental faculties. Scarlett, do you know where you are?"

Scarlett, her voice becoming stronger, said, "Barnett Center."

"What year is it?" said Ansley.

"2042," said Scarlett, her voice now clear and strong.

"Are you feeling any pain or discomfort?"

"No. I thought I would not feel pain in this body," said Scarlett.

Ansley, pleased with Scarlett's progress and apparent mental awareness, said, "that's not entirely true. You will not feel pain in the human sense, but your synthetic body will warn you via an electronic signal when you encounter a condition that could damage it. The signal will be like being shocked by a low voltage electrical current."

"Ansley, her finger moved!" exclaimed Savannah. "Scarlett, keep trying to move your left appendages."

Scarlett moved one finger first, then partially closed her fingers into a fist and then relaxed her fist.

"Excellent!" said Ansley. Now try to move your toes.

After several seconds, the big toe on her left foot twitched.

"Keep trying, Scarlett," said Savannah.

After moving her toe several times, Scarlett could move all of her toes and move her foot from side to side.

Testing her new body continued for several weeks following Scarlett's transition to her synthetic body. At first, progress was slow as Scarlett learned to control her artificial body. About three weeks were required for her to learn to walk comfortably and it was several more weeks before she could run with confidence that she would not lose her balance. In addition, Scarlett had to learn how to control her hands, including how to grip eating utensils and how to write. Typing on a keyboard was especially challenging at first, as it had been with the other three cyborgs after transitioning to their synthetic bodies. Even though typing on a keyboard had only been required for specialized scientific and engineering applications by 2042, it was considered an excellent exercise to improve the cyborg's dexterity. Finally, getting used to the strength of her synthetic body was also a challenge. During tennis lessons with Savannah, Scarlett sent the ball through the fence bordering the court behind Savannah, shredding its cover and breaking the strings on her racquet. Per orders direct from SecDef, military cyborgs' strength was not to be limited artificially. Erik Richards had cautioned her he was still learning to control his strength when in public and that he had experienced a couple of instances where his true strength was exposed.

Chapter Five

October 14, 2042, 9:10 AM. Erik's smartphone buzzed, indicating he had received a text message. He was sitting in the office of Captain Jeffrey Barnes, his commanding officer, to discuss the possibility of informing Ksenia Anderson, with whom Erik had developed a relationship, of his transition to a synthetic body. Erik ignored the text message, thinking he would retrieve it after the meeting.

"Jeff, I need to make you aware that Ksenia and my relationship is growing and becoming serious," said Erik. "I am considering proposing to her soon, but I want to inform her of my… condition before I do."

"Erik, you know the conditions that you agreed to when you were selected for the transformation. I do not believe SecDef, nor DARPA will be in favor of informing Ksenia without a need to know."

"Begging your pardon, sir, but wouldn't the woman I am asking to spend the rest of her life with me need to know? With your support, I could make a request to SecDef to consider allowing me to inform her."

"Erik, if I am correct, you can fulfill your vows as a husband without her knowing."

"Yes, physically I can, but how do I explain my need to plug in to recharge this body regularly? I doubt I could hide that activity for very long."

Pondering Erik's argument for a moment, Captain Barnes said, "Draft a letter to me requesting to inform Ksenia of your intentions with her and why you believe it is necessary to inform her of your condition. I will pass it up the chain and see where it lands."

"Thank you, sir," said Erik, rising to leave the captain's office.

Back in his office, Erik recalled he had received a text video message. He laid his smartphone down on its charger and a six-inch-tall holographic image of Ksenia, dressed in her Viking Cruise Lines uniform, appeared above it saying, "I have left the ship and am on my way to the airport in Venice. I will fly to Bergen today to complete my cruise and depart tomorrow, Wednesday, for the U.S. My flight is United 243 and scheduled to arrive at 3:25 PM local time. Can you meet me at the airport?"

Even the low-resolution holographic images of Ksenia arrested Erik's attention when he saw them, and it quickly dawned on him he was just staring and smiling. "Reply," commanded Erik to his smartphone. "Yes, I will meet you at the airport. I can't wait to see you!" Erik then texted Captain Barnes. "I will need to leave the office tomorrow by about 1415 hours to meet Ksenia arriving at Dulles. Before I leave, you will have the letter on your desk. Thanks."

Erik then drafted the letter that he hoped would find its way to SecDef's attention.

Erik walked through the door of the international arrivals terminal at Dulles International Airport at 3:05 PM, October 15, 2042. He tapped his smartphone and said, "status of United 243 arriving from Bergen."

The smartphone's AI responded, "United Airlines Flight 243 is estimating touchdown at Dulles at 1531 hours. Anticipated arrival time of passengers in baggage claim is 1615 hours." Erik's clocks and watch were set to 24-hour military time.

Erik proceeded towards the exit of the immigration hall and did some casual window shopping along the way. As he approached a gift store, he realized he had gotten nothing to give to Ksenia when she arrived. He went into the gift store, desperately looking for a small token that would express his feelings about seeing Ksenia after her three-month cruise. He saw a young woman standing behind a glass jewelry counter and walked up to her, saying, "I need some help. I have someone arriving in a few minutes and need a small gift for her."

The young woman looked up at Erik and immediately got lost in his azure blue eyes. "Oh, yes," she said after regaining her composure. "Is this gift for your wife, girlfriend, mom?"

"My, uh, girlfriend. I need something small, like earrings or a necklace."

"Let me see. Hmmm, how about these tiny earrings?" she said, pointing to the pair near the front of the cabinet. "They are plumeria flowers made of platinum and opal. Very delicate."

"Perfect. Can you gift wrap them?" he said after a quick glance at the earring.

"Don't you want to know how much they cost?" said the young woman.

"OK. How much?"

"Four-hundred thirty-nine dollars," she responded, timidly.

"I'll take them. Can you gift wrap them?"

"Sure. It will just take me a few minutes. I'll be right back," she said as she walked into a room behind the counter.

"Thanks, please hurry!" said Erik.

In a few minutes, the saleswoman emerged from the back office with the earrings wrapped in white paper with silver embroidery. "How's this?" she said to Erik.

"Perfect!"

"Here's the price tag. Please hold your smartphone close to pay." A split-second later, Erik's smartphone beeped, showing the payment had been made, which would be charged to his personal American Express credit account. He turned and exited the gift shop, heading towards baggage claim, thinking to himself, "Nice catch, Erik. I would have looked like… like a rube showing up empty-handed."

Erik stood near the exit from the immigration and customs hall, watching passengers meet their loved ones waiting for them. After what seemed like hours but was only about ten minutes, he saw Ksenia. At that moment, all their cares dissolved as they just smiled at each other. She hurried towards Erik with her baggage in tow. He thought she looked like an angel coming from heaven.

Erik embraced her, lifting her off the floor with no thought of caution regarding his synthetic strength. She let out a woosh of air in surprise while he quickly recovered from his unplanned display of strength.

"I thought for a moment that you were going to throw me back into customs," said Ksenia, smiling, as Erik extended his arms, releasing her.

"I am just so happy to have you here!" he said. "You made it through immigration and customs quickly. I need to learn your tricks for doing that."

"Well, if you are able, pick the immigration station with the most normal looking people waiting in line. Businesspeople, families with children, older couples. Most CBP (Customs and Border Patrol) agents are bored with these people and process them through quickly by asking just a few questions. I also try to pick stations manned by men. That way, I can try to flirt a little, which makes me appear both harmless and vulnerable. That usually works well. But if I get stuck with a woman agent, many of them give me stern looks as if I must be guilty of something and often ask detailed questions regarding my stay."

"I just got a text message saying our Uber car is ready. Let's get out of here," said Erik.

Erik held the door to the backseat of the self-navigating Uber car as Ksenia hopped in, then walked around to the other door and got in. He then held his smartphone up to the scanner hanging off the back of the car's front seat and gave the address of their destination. The driverless car then merged into traffic and exited the airport on the Dulles Access Road and on to Arlington to his apartment near the Pentagon.

"Oh, I almost forgot," said Erik, reaching into his uniform jacket pocket. "Here's a little something to welcome you back," handing the small square gift box to Ksenia.

For a moment, Ksenia seemed stunned. The gift box looked very much like one that would contain an engagement ring and its white and gold wrapping looked like wedding gift paper. She removed the wrapping paper slowly, revealing a blue box. She unconsciously held her breath as she opened the box and then breathed a quiet sigh of relief when she saw the delicate earrings inside. "These are beautiful, Erik," she said as she leaned over and kissed him. "Thank you."

"I hoped you would like them. They just seemed like... you. Beautiful, delicate but strong," he said.

They arrived at Erik's apartment about thirty minutes later. Immediately after entering the apartment and closing the door, they embraced, kissing passionately. Kissing soon turned to more sensuous foreplay and in no time, they were removing each other's clothes as they moved towards the bedroom. There, they made love until Ksenia fell asleep in Erik's arms. Erik just lay there with a smile on his face, with even greater certainty that he wanted to spend the rest of his life with her.

Chapter Six

Friday, November 14, 2042.

"Yes, sir," said Erik, standing in the doorway to Captain Jeffrey Barnes' office.

"Come in, Erik, and have a seat," said Captain Barnes, sitting behind the standard Navy issue metal desk. Barnes' rank entitled him to an office with a window which was directly behind the desk. "I have received a request to send you to the Barnett Center for Neurological Restoration. Lt. Scarlett Bross has requested your help, and Drs. Barnett and Richards concur. Please travel to The Center as soon as possible. From the communique sent to me by the doctors, you may need to stay out there for several weeks. While there, I expect you to continue working on the starship project as much as possible."

"I have also received a response to your request from SecDef. Here is a hard copy of the response," said Barnes, handing a single sheet of paper to Erik.

"Commander Richards, while we can appreciate your desire to share your condition with the person you envision becoming your spouse, we cannot release you from your obligation to keep your condition top secret. If for any reason the relationship fails after disclosure to Ms. Anderson, there remains the possibility that your condition could be exposed to the public. We hope you will understand the position of the United States and we wish you success in both your personal and professional life." Signed William H. Bonner, Secretary of Defense

"Well, this is certainly disappointing," said Erik after a pause of several seconds. "I still believe it would be unfair to Ksenia to keep my condition hidden from her. If I wait to disclose my condition to her until after we're married, I'm afraid it would destroy her trust in me. I will need to give this situation some serious thought. Thank you, Captain, for going to bat for me."

Erik returned to his office and called Ksenia, who was staying with him at his apartment.

"Hello, Erik," said Ksenia. "Can we meet for lunch?"

"Yes, yes," said Erik. "But I need you to pack. We will travel to Barnett Center this evening. It seems my sister and Ansley, Dr. Barnett, want me to… work with a naval aviator who was injured and is recovering at the Center. The aviator is receiving the same type of care that I received during my recovery. I will text you the flight information once my virtual assistant arranges it."

"So, I will meet your sister?" asked Ksenia, thinking she will need to pick out her best outfits. "Is there anything I should do to make a good impression on her?"

"Just be yourself and you will do fine," said Erik, smiling at the nervousness he detected in Ksenia's voice.

Later that evening, Erik and Ksenia arrived at LAX and were greeted by a chauffeur in the baggage claim area holding a tablet displaying COMMANDER ERIK RICHARDS in large white letters on a black background. "Commander Richards?" said the chauffeur as Erik and Ksenia walked up to her.

"Yes, said Erik. You will take us to Barnett Center?"

"Yes. My name is Julie. Do you have checked baggage to claim?"

"Yes, three bags. I will go wait for them to come down to the carousel."

"No, need, Commander. I will get your bags. You and the lady can proceed to my limo just outside the door to your right. Black Chevy Tahoe, License plate is BRNET5.”

“You get a chauffeur?” said Ksenia, briefly laughing, as they walked out to the limo.

“Nothing but the best for one of the center’s star patients,” said Erik, also laughing.

In about ten minutes, Julie exited the terminal and loaded their baggage in the back of the SUV. She entered the driver’s side of the vehicle, pushed a button to start the electric engine, and verbally gave the destination to the vehicle’s autopilot. The navigation system then synced with the Los Angeles area traffic system, and they slowly pulled into traffic, heading for the airport exit. The trip from LAX to Barnett Center in Bel Air took twenty-eight minutes.

As the vehicle entered the Barnett Center grounds, Julie said, “I am told that you will stay in one of the Center’s guesthouses.” The SUV pulled up to an attractive, quaint redwood and stone bungalow designed to blend in nicely with the surrounding foliage. All three exited the vehicle, and Julie opened the tailgate and unloaded the baggage.

“Thank you, Julie. You’ve been very helpful,” said Erik as he offered Julie a $50 tip.

“Oh, no thank you, sir,” said Julie. “Barnett chauffeurs do not accept tips.”

“You sure?” said Erik, smiling. “We won’t tell anyone.”

“I really can’t accept it, sir,” said Julie, smiling. “It’s been a pleasure serving you this evening.” She turned to get back into the SUV.

Erik grabbed Ksenia’s two bags, and they entered the front door of the guesthouse together. He then returned to the drive and got his bag. The house was twenty-three hundred square feet with an open great room with kitchen, and two master bedrooms. The furnishings were all coordinated hardwoods. The great room was furnished with two teal leather recliners and a leather sofa. A large, round glass coffee table sat in the middle of the floor next to the seating. At the rear of the great room, a triple slider opened on to a lanai, complete with an outdoor kitchen and swimming pool.

"Very nice," said Ksenia, as they stepped out onto the lanai. "I think we will be quite comfortable here."

"Yes, it is nice. But wait until you see the Barnett Mansion," said Erik, pointing to the enormous structure up the hill to the north. "It is what I would call a true American castle."

"I really should unpack. Let's check out the bedrooms and see which one we want," said Ksenia.

"I think we should make love in each before deciding," said Erik, grabbing Ksenia around the waist as they walked to the bedroom where they had placed their baggage.

The next morning, Erik dressed casually in a navy-blue golf shirt bearing a Top Gun insignia over his left breast, and khakis. He walked to the Center on the one-third mile winding pathway next to a garden to meet with Ansley, Savannah and Scarlett while Ksenia stayed at the guesthouse. When he arrived at the Center, he checked in at reception and proceeded to the fourth floor, where Ansley's and Savannah's offices were housed. He continued to Savannah's office.

"Morning, sis," Erik said as he stood in the open doorway, smiling. "How are you this fine California morning?"

"Erik, Hi, so great to see my spaceman brother!" said Savannah, rising to come from behind the desk to exchange a hug. "You look terrific. I believe Ksenia is contributing to your health. How is she?"

"Right now, I believe she is sleeping in at the bungalow. And yes, she is definitely boosting my spirits."

"Any… plans on the wedding front?" said Savannah.

"Well, to be honest, I believe Ksenia is definitely the 'one'. But, given my condition, it is complicated. Perhaps we could have some time for me to get some sisterly advice later?"

"Sure. Absolutely. After all, what are sisters for but to help their brothers in romantic situations? I believe it is time for our meeting with Scarlett. We're meeting just down the hall in the executive conference room."

Chapter Seven

Ansley and Scarlett Bross were seated in the conference room when Savannah and Erik entered. Also present were Dr. Samuel McKensey, Head of Psychiatry at the Barnett Center, and Aaron Adams, who was the first human transitioned to an artificial body.

"Good morning, Erik and Savannah. Please join us. I believe everyone here knows everyone. The reason we are here this morning is to review Scarlett's progress transitioning to her artificial body and to address any concerns she may have. Scarlett is making excellent progress. Scarlett, do you have any comments before we begin?"

"Thank you, Dr. Barnett. First, I want to express my sincere gratitude for the opportunity to replace my severely damaged human body with this miracle of science and technology," said Scarlett, motioning her hands to point at herself. "I also want to thank Drs. Richards, Barnett, and McKensey for their amazing dedication to my full recovery as a cyborg. However, I have some concerns that may affect my… adjustment to my new existence," said Scarlett as she then hesitated while observing reactions by the others in the room.

"Go on, Scarlett," said Ansley.

"Well, I feel that with this body, that I am considered more an experiment than a person. I hope that what Dr. McKensey told me, that once I leave full-time residence at the Center, those feelings will pass. People that see me then won't know I am… artificial."

"Erik, Aaron, did you experience similar concerns during your recovery from the transition while here at the Center?" asked Ansley.

"I suspect that the feelings and emotions one experiences during the transition and recovery process will differ for each individual," said Aaron. "I was so happy to regain the use of a functioning body, I did not experience any concerns with how people saw me. My early thoughts were along the lines of what happens if this body fails. But as I grew more confident in my ability to control my artificial body, those concerns faded away."

"Before the transition, I was suffering from severe depression," confessed Erik. "All I could do was lie in bed and breathe. I had no control of body functions, little movement in one arm. My spine had been nearly destroyed, beyond even the Center's advanced spinal recovery program's recovery protocols. My career was over. My life was essentially over. So, after transition, I too was elated and treated the adjustment to my new body as a challenge that I was going to meet. Post-transition, I did not experience any of the concerns Scarlett has expressed. And I have established a very close and personal relationship with Ksenia, who suspects nothing after several months."

"What are your other concerns, Scarlett?" asked Ansley.

"I am concerned that I will not be viewed as a woman capable of a close romantic relationship when I am ready, and the right person comes along. I know Erik has expressed that he has done exactly that with no problem. But, Erik, what happens when you are ready to take the next step with Ksenia? Are you going to tell her about your… condition, should you both decide that marriage is a possibility?"

"Interesting that you raise that question, Scarlett," said Erik. "I have requested release of my obligation of secrecy regarding Ksenia," carefully stopping there so as not to upset Scarlett with the response he received from SecDef. "But, Scarlett, you have transitioned. You are now a cyborg. Do not allow yourself to succumb to emotions over which you currently have little control. Concentrate instead on taking complete command of this miracle you've been given."

"Going back to your perception that we're looking at you like you are some kind of experiment," said Ansley. "What if Erik was to assume supervision of your training? Would you have a problem with that? After all, you're both naval aviators and have experienced challenging training regimens since you entered flight training."

"I would be OK with that if Erik wanted to do it. But that decision may not be his alone to make. Would his command agree to a temporary reassignment?"

"His command has already agreed that, if we believed his involvement in your recovery is necessary, he could be assigned temporarily."

Chapter Eight

Later that evening, Scarlett was lying on her recharging bed, thinking about Erik taking over her cyborg transition program. She had only just met Erik and knew little about him, aside from what she had been told by Ansley and Savannah. But, she thought, they had a lot in common. Both were naval aviators that strived to be on top of their game one hundred percent of the time. They competed at a level where there is no reward for second place.

After an unknown amount of time, Scarlett's mind relaxed, and she fell into the neo-sleep state common to the cyborgs, whose synthetic bodies needed no rest in the human sense. As she lay on her back, motionless on the recharging bed with its cable attached to the base of her skull enabling the backup of her mind and charging the batteries in her synthetic body, she saw a mist form. As the mist grew thicker, she saw a shape form. The shape slowly formed into that of a man, and as it became clearer, she saw a man dressed in a white t-shirt, blue jeans, motorcycle boots, with a long leather coat and a Stetson. Long, curly blond locks fell from underneath the Stetson.

"Scarlett, do not be alarmed. I will not harm you and you are in no danger. I have come to enlist you for missions to save humanity and the world in which you exist. You, your spiritual being or soul, has been separated from your human body. Normally, this separation is called death by humans, and the spirit ascends to an immortal state of pure energy. But in your case, and the case of others whom I call, you cannot ascend to the next level of existence. Your spirit is bound to the synthetic body that it occupies."

"Am… am I dreaming this?" said Scarlett, a tinge of panic in her voice and her hands open in front of her as she sat up on the bed, still connected to the charging cable. "Who are you, and what do you want with me?"

"No, you are not dreaming, Scarlett. Others like you call me Guardian. I am one of those beings that humans have referred to as an angel throughout much of history. The image of me you see puts humans at ease, especially the first time they see me. If you were to see my true appearance, you would likely be driven insane and perhaps blinded." The Guardian then emitted a golden glow around his body for a few seconds to confirm what he had told Scarlett, who remained shocked and speechless.

"Do you have questions?" said The Guardian.

Scarlett thought for a few moments, then said, "What is your… your purpose? How am I involved with your purpose?"

"The reason your colleagues call me Guardian is I am charged by The Creator to watch timelines. When timelines go awry and threaten a free human existence, I go to that time and make efforts to correct the errant timeline. The ability to enlist the support of human minds is a recent development that provides much greater strength and opportunity to keep Evil at bay in its never-ending attempts to destroy the soul of humanity."

"Why can't you use the minds of people that have fully… ascended to the next state of existence?"

"Once a human spirit fully ascends, it cannot return to the corporeal plane of existence. Since you have not fully ascended, you can exist on both planes, the higher plane, for short periods of time. This provides you, your spirit, with the ability to travel to other time periods with my help."

"So… what timelines have you been able to correct since enlisting the support of… people like me?"

"Several, all of which would have been disastrous for humanity had they not been corrected. In fact, none of what you see around you would exist had we not corrected even one timeline. The outcome of the U.S. Civil War, World War II, and The Cuban Missile Crisis are just a few of the timelines that had to be corrected."

"When will you call on me to join you on a… mission?" asked Scarlett.

"Soon, there is a timeline in 2020 that is showing signs of manipulation by evil that could destroy the United States as you know it." With that, The Guardian faded into a mist until both he and the mist disappeared. Shortly, Scarlett opened her eyes, fully awake, wondering what she had just seen. Had it been a dream? If so, it was the most realistic dream she had ever experienced. Then she realized she may have heard confirmation that there is an afterlife. Raised as a Christian, she had always believed in an afterlife, but to hear it confirmed by a supernatural being was incredible. She made herself a mental note to ask The Guardian more about the afterlife when he returned.

Chapter Nine

It was Tuesday, November 18, 2042, 0915. Erik and Scarlett met on the outdoor track at the Barnett Center's gym complex. "Good morning, Scarlett," said Erik. "Let's start out with a couple of slow laps around the track to warm up."

"Hi Erik. Good idea," said Scarlett, as the two began jogging. "Erik, have you experienced any… strange dreams since you transitioned?"

"What do you mean by strange dreams?" he replied. "While recharging, I try to relax and let my mind wander wherever it wants. I can now enter a sleep-like state of consciousness that seems to refresh my mind and maintain my alertness."

"Yes, I can usually do that, too. But I am talking about lifelike dreams. Dreams where you are in a… conversation with another. Dreams that are more like visions you do not forget."

"To be quite honest, yes, I have experienced dreams like you describe. Tell me about your dream and we will see if it is like what I have experienced," said Erik.

"Last night, as I lay on the recharging bed and had fallen into a deep state of rest, I had a dream, a vision. The vision started as a thick mist and quickly formed into that of a man dressed like something you would see in an old western film. He referred to himself as Guardian and said his purpose was to correct timelines in the past that had gone astray, threatening humanity."

"Let me guess," said Erik. "The Guardian then described himself, and the role that we who've transitioned have supporting his missions?"

"Yes!" said Scarlett. "So, you have had this… experience. Is The Guardian for real? Has he taken you with him on a mission?"

"Oh yeah!" exclaimed Erik. "He is most definitely for real. So far, I've been on one mission that possibly corrected the annihilation of the world in a nuclear holocaust. Let's pickup the pace on the next lap."

"Tell me about that mission, Erik. What was your role? What was The Guardian's role?"

"This is where it gets… complicated. We cyborgs not only time travel with The Guardian, but our minds can also influence, even control, the minds of others. We can take possession of their minds and affect outcomes without their knowledge. This is often how errant timelines are corrected."

"This is sounding weird. You actually took possession of someone's mind?

"Yes," said Erik. "The mission was to correct the timeline for the Cuban Missile Crisis in the early 1960s. The U.S. and the Soviet Union came very close to nuclear war during that period. The U.S.S.R. began placing nuclear-tipped missiles in Cuba. The U.S. objected and implemented a blockade around Cuba to prevent the delivery of the missiles. My role was to fly a sortie with a Navy pilot across Cuba at low altitude to observe and photograph a missile site under construction. It was actually fun to fly in one of those antique fighters. Of course, I was in spirit form, undetectable to the pilot, and took up no visible space in the aircraft. We took machine gun ground fire as we flew over the missile site, but nothing critical was damaged. When we returned to NAS Key West, the pilot, Commander William Ecker, was immediately summoned to Washington D.C. to meet with the Joint Chiefs. When the question asked of Ecker by General LeMay–'were you shot at by as much as a BB gun flying over Cuba?'–I took possession of Ecker's mind and said, 'No, it was a walk in the park.' The meeting then ended. I left Ecker's mind and left Ecker wondering where that expression had come from. My response on Ecker's behalf to the Joint Chiefs apparently diffused their intention to attack and invade Cuba."

"For this last lap, let's fire up our afterburners and go all out," said Erik. The conversation stopped at this point until the end of their run.

Erik completed the quarter-mile loop in thirty-one seconds while Scarlett, who stumbled twice, took forty-three seconds. To compare their performance, consider the fastest mile run by a human is just under four minutes.

"Not bad for a newbie," said Erik. "Any trouble with your legs? It looks like you stumbled a bit when we started."

"I think I am still getting used to controlling these artificial legs… and this artificial body," said Scarlett. "I feel great and believe I just need a bit more practice."

"How about we try playing some tennis?" said Erik. "Tennis is a great way to learn how to control your arm strength and speed so that you don't accidentally look superhuman in public."

"Sounds good," said Scarlett as they began walking back to the clubhouse to get tennis gear.

"Better grab two racquets. You'll probably break the strings on the first one you use."

As they were walking out to the tennis court, Scarlett said, "When I first met you, you said you were in a relationship. Not meaning to get too personal, but are you still in that relationship?"

"Yes, and we are growing closer. I am considering proposing to her soon. Would you like to meet Ksenia? She is here at the Center with me during her leave from Viking."

"… Yes," said Scarlett, momentarily hesitating while thinking Erik sure was a hunk. He can mesmerize me with his beautiful eyes.

"Great, I will set up a dinner out for the three of us."

After stepping onto the tennis court, Erik and Scarlett began volleying back and forth across the net. The first time Scarlett had to run and reach to hit a backhand, she broke the strings on the racquet and sent the ball through the chain-link fence at the back of the baseline, stripping its cover, which was still stuck in the fence.

"See, I told you that you would need a second racquet. Now concentrate on controlling your newfound strength," said Erik. "I know it is difficult because I let down my control twice in public and almost blew my cover. But it is critical that we do not indulge our superhuman strength in public settings. The media would explode if they saw us."

After approximately one hour of play, they left the tennis court and began walking back to the Center's gym complex when Scarlett said, "So, you are thinking about proposing to Ksenia. If you love her as much as you say, what is holding you back?"

"As you know, we are under strict non-disclosure of our... condition to persons not approved by SecDef. I wrote a letter to SecDef stating my intentions towards Ksenia and requesting approval to disclose my condition to her. He denied the request, stating that I could not tell her about my situation until after we've wed. My concern, that I also expressed, is that waiting until after we're married to share something that important would destroy her trust in me."

"Wow, that would really piss me off," replied Scarlett. "I understand the military has given us a new, incredible life. But now they expect us to sacrifice any opportunity to have a normal relationship? I will write to SecDef myself and express my concern on your behalf. This is simply ridiculous!"

"Whoa, please don't do that! It could end badly for both of us if you do," said Erik.

"I will be respectful and write the letter from a perspective of a woman seeking advice rather than attacking SecDef's decision."

"I still don't believe it will be a good idea to do so. You know as well as I do, the Navy doesn't condone questioning policy by those in the rank and file."

"But we need to get this... policy taken care of now. If I develop a serious relationship with someone, I want to share everything with him. I will give it more thought, but I am very concerned," said Scarlett.

Chapter Ten

Erik returned to the guest cottage to have lunch and spend the afternoon working on his starship project. "Hi, Ksenia," he said as he walked to where she was reading out on the lanai. "I think they stocked the fridge with cold-cuts and there's fresh bread in the pantry. Can I make you a sandwich?"

"Sure. How was your morning with Scarlett?"

"Interesting. She is coming along well with her… rehabilitation." Erik hated the secrecy surrounding the cyborg program when speaking with Ksenia. Also, he hated keeping information from her regarding the starship project that was also classified Top Secret.

As they sat down at the round wrought-iron table on the lanai to eat, he received a written text on his smartphone from his boss at the Pentagon, Captain Barnes. "Make plans to meet the project team at Groom Lake on 2 December. Stay will be 2-3 days. Call me to discuss details."

"Who is that from?" asked Ksenia.

"Captain Barnes. I will need to go to Arizona for a few days after Thanksgiving to meet on the project I'm working on."

"What project is that?" said Ksenia.

"Sorry, hon, that's classified. Remember that I told you that the project was more important than my return to space?"

"I suppose so…," said Ksenia. "I hate being kept in the dark regarding your work."

"I hate it too, but I'm afraid it comes with the job. I would share it with you if I could."

"Don't you trust me enough to keep your secrets?" she said, displaying a playful fake pout with her lower lip extended.

Erik, taking her question a little more seriously, said, "Oh, I trust you. But what if you were kidnapped and held hostage, even tortured, to give up information? Maybe given truth serum to make you spill the beans?"

"Then I think you would rescue me before that happened," she said playfully.

After lunch, they changed and went for a dip in the swimming pool. Friendly horseplay quickly turned into serious foreplay, which resulted in the two heading for the shower. As the hot water poured over them, they made love, each caressing the other in streams of water and soap.

Afterward, as they were dressing, Erik said, "I'd like for you to meet Scarlett. How about dinner on Thursday? I'll get a recommendation for a restaurant from Savannah. I think getting out for an evening would be good for Scarlett's rehab. From my experience, sitting around alone every night when I was rehabilitating got quite old."

Ksenia hesitated for a moment, then said, "Well, if you think it is best, I could go for an evening out." She had a moment of concern, thinking that Erik was spending his day with Scarlett… but then discarded the thought.

Chapter Eleven

Erik, Ksenia, and Scarlett arrived at Vibrato, a Bel Air restaurant recommended by Savannah, a few minutes before their reservation for 7:30 PM, Thursday, November 20, 2042. They were seated immediately.

"Scarlett, Erik told me you were injured seriously trying to land your plane on an aircraft carrier. You look amazing after such a terrible experience. What's the secret to your quick recovery?"

"Thanks, Ksenia. I must admit that I did not know about the advanced medical technology that exists at Barnett Center. After my accident, I never thought I would walk again, much less return to flying. Now, with Erik pushing me through my rehab, flying again is within reach," said Scarlett, looking briefly at Erik.

A young woman dressed in a light blue blouse, dark blue skirt, and low-heeled black pumps approached their table. "Hello, my name is Emily, and I will be your server this evening. Welcome to Vibrato. Can I get you a cocktail?

Looking at the list of specialty cocktails, Ksenia said with a short giggle, "Yes, I think I will try the Skinny Dip." Erik glanced at her and smiled.

"And you, miss?" said Emily to Scarlett.

"I think I'll just have a glass of the David Marchesi Napa Chardonnay 2019. I need to take it easy. This will be the first alcohol I've had since the accident," said Scarlett, knowing that alcohol would have no effect on her synthetic body, but that anything stronger may raise Ksenia's eyebrows.

"And you, sir?" said Emily.

"Yes, I would like a Glenfiddich 15-Year-Old Solera Reserve Single Malt Scotch Whisky on the rocks," said Erik.

"Thank you," said Emily. "I will be back shortly with your drinks."

"So, Scarlett, how is your rehab going?" asked Ksenia. "I hope Erik isn't being overly demanding."

"Erik seems to know how far he can push me. But then, pushes harder. Sometimes I think he's just trying to be like his drill instructors at the academy," Scarlett said, smiling at Erik, which didn't go unnoticed by Ksenia.

"Hey, be careful or I'll drill you like a plebe, Lieutenant," said Erik, laughing before realizing his statement could be wrongly interpreted. He then blushed and looked at Ksenia, who was drilling him with her eyes.

Emily returned with their drinks and said, "Are we ready to order?"

"Let's order an appetizer while we take a longer look at the menu. I suggest an order of crab cakes and lamb lollipops. Ladies, anything else that you'd like?" Ksenia and Scarlett showed they were good with Erik's recommendation with a brief wave.

"Great choices, sir. The lollipops are my favorite! I will put this in right away and should have it out to you quickly," said Emily.

Ksenia then asked Scarlett, "How did you decide you wanted to fly fighter jets for the Navy?"

"As a kid growing up, I was a tomboy. I usually played with boys in the neighborhood trying to do the things boys do, beating them at their own games often. I climbed trees, was into skateboarding, went fishing in the river behind our house. A neighbor yelled at me to get down from the tree that I climbed. She was panicking since I'd climbed higher than the boys I was with. I took martial arts classes for several years, earning my Black Belt and competing against boys. I took flying lessons and soloed on my sixteenth birthday. That is when I knew then that I wanted a career in aviation."

"Hey, I soloed on my sixteenth birthday," said Erik.

"What made you decide to go into the Navy?" asked Ksenia.

"I started investigating the military academies to get my education and achieve a career in aviation. For me, the Navy seemed to offer the greatest challenge. I still believe shooting touch and goes on an aircraft carrier deck is among the most challenging flying there is. I applied to Annapolis and was accepted. I believe I entered my plebe year the same year that Erik graduated, but I don't recall having met him then. How about you, Ksenia? How did you decide on a sea-going career?"

Emily returned with the appetizers. "Are you ready to order your main course?"

"I think so," said Erik. "Ladies?"

"Yes, I will have The Madame, cooked medium," said Ksenia, which was a 6 oz. petite filet with shoestring truffle fries.

"I would like the Ora King Salmon," said Scarlett.

"Sir?" said Emily.

"I'll have the Cowboy, medium rare," said Erik. Which was a twenty-four-ounce bone in ribeye. "Also, the loaded baked potato."

"Anything else to drink?"

"Water with lime for me," said Scarlett.

"Ksenia, share a bottle of wine with me?" said Erik.

"That would be lovely."

"A bottle of Prime Coombs Ville Napa Valley Cabernet, please," said Erik.

"Very good, sir," said Emily, turning and walking away from the table.

"I'm surprised you didn't order the Norwegian halibut, Ksenia," said Erik.

"I think we're too far away for Norwegian fish the way I know it," said Ksenia.

"Scarlett, back to your last question. When I was twelve, we moved from Sweden to Norway, to an estate that was left to my mother. From the property, we could see down into the fjord where the cruise ships would dock in the summer months. From the first time I saw one of those beautiful ships, I knew I wanted to have a maritime career."

"How did you pursue your career? What did you do to prepare for that career?" asked Scarlett.

"In my third year of high school, I began researching maritime schools. The United States Merchant Marine Academy was one of the top schools for merchant crews. I applied through our foreign service bureau and was accepted by Kings Point. I was able to spend my sea year at the academy on cruise ships and cargo ships and returned to secure a position with Viking Cruise Lines."

"A toast to the three academy grads at this table tonight," said Erik, raising his glass.

The three finished dinner and returned to Barnett Center. Erik and Ksenia walked to the guest cottage. Ksenia was silent for the length of the ten-minute walk.

When they entered the cottage, Erik said, "What did you think of Scarlett?"

"She seems genuinely nice, and quite determined. I believe one would have to be… determined to do what she is doing. I also sense that she and you have a good working relationship that seems to be growing."

"Growing? What do you mean by growing?"

"Growing into… one of friendship… or beyond, perhaps?"

"Beyond friendship? What are you getting at, Ksenia?

"I could sense that there is more to your relationship than, shall we say, professional? The glances you shared hinted at something… more between you two. Do you find her attractive?"

Erik sensed Ksenia was becoming more emotional as her Norwegian accent became more pronounced. "She is an attractive woman. I won't deny that, but that doesn't mean that she is something more than a professional colleague to me."

"Will she be accompanying you on your trip to Arizona next month?"

"No. Scarlett is not involved in any of my assignments other than her rehabilitation program. Where are you going with this, Ksenia? Are you doubting my feelings for you?"

"I don't know," said Ksenia, as she turned and walked towards the lanai.

Erik followed her and said, "Look, I have fallen in love with you. I've told you that and it hasn't changed. My love for you grows every day. Someday, I hope you will join me as my wife. That is how strongly I care for you." It was the first time Erik mentioned the possibility of marriage.

Ksenia stopped and turned around to face Erik, tears swelling in her eyes. "Do you mean that? Don't say that to me if you do not mean it," her accent growing even more pronounced.

Erik approached Ksenia and took her shoulders firmly but gently in his hands. "Ksenia, I mean every word. I believe now that fate brought us together for a reason. I have no romantic intentions toward Scarlett or any other woman. I don't want any other woman. I want to be with you. But for that to happen, we must trust each other. Do you think you can trust me?"

Ksenia looked into Erik's eyes and saw that he was being sincere. "Yes, I trust you."

The two then hugged as they walked to the bedroom when Erik received a written text message from Ansley.

"Thanksgiving celebration at the mansion. Can you and Ksenia come?"

Erik then said to Ksenia, "We've been invited to Barnett Mansion for Thanksgiving. Wanna go?"

"How could we turn that down? Sure, I've been wanting to see an American borg (Norwegian for castle). Oh my, I brought nothing suitable to wear for such an event. I'll need to do some shopping!"

"Ksenia, you're in California. They are very informal here. I'll probably wear a golf shirt and blue jeans. You'd be out-of-place dressing formal."

Erik confirmed their attendance in a reply to Ansley's text, "Great! We'll be there. Thanks, Ansley."

The next day, Ksenia went shopping and mostly ignored Erik's recommendation on attire for their visit to the mansion. She picked out a couple of chic outfits, including a couple pairs of shoes.

Chapter Twelve

Thanksgiving, November 27, 2042.

Shortly past noon, Ksenia and Erik walked from the guest cottage to the Center and took the escalator from the first floor down to the transporter lobby. Erik wore a light blue golf shirt with a logo of the USS Elon Musk on the left breast, blue jeans, and Sperry boat shoes. Ksenia wore one of the casual outfits, skorts and a sleeveless top under a sweater that she purchased a few days before.

The transporter was a hyperloop that connected the Center with the mansion. They boarded a transporter car and were whisked to the mansion in under five seconds. The transporter hyperloop technology was a product of Barnett Industries and was installed in many cities globally. In the U.S. it connected several cities including Los Angeles with San Francisco and Las Vegas with stops at each city's international airport, Boston-New York-Washington, D.C., Dallas and Fort Worth, with a stop at DFW, and Tampa-Orlando-Daytona Beach-Jacksonville and Palm Beach-Ft. Lauderdale-Miami, including stops at Tampa International Airport, Orlando International Airport, and Miami International Airport. Where the system had been deployed, it had virtually eliminated short-distance commercial air traffic and much vehicle traffic, reducing greenhouse emissions.

In the mansion's transporter lobby, they exited their car and rode up the escalator to the main lobby, where they were greeted by Miquel, the mansion facility and security manager. "Good morning, Commander, Miss Anderson. If you will follow me, I will take you to the other guests." They boarded an elevator and Miquel said, "pool deck."

"I believe that the chandelier in the lobby is the largest I've ever seen," said Ksenia. "And the wall coverings are exquisite."

They reached the pool deck level quickly and exited to see Kristian, Ansley, Savannah, and Aaron standing together at the far end of the pool. They also saw young Kristen Elaine, Kristian and Ansley's daughter, now seven years old, playing in the shallow end of the heated pool.

The pool deck spanned the entire top level of the mansion. The pool was a rectangular infinity pool and had a slide and wave machine that was installed for Kristen Elaine. It also featured a current generating machine to use for swimming exercise. There were several round redwood tables with umbrellas, redwood deck chairs and loungers with ornate pillows containing images of Southern California beach and boating scenes depicting life in the 1950s. Next to the pool was a hot tub that could accommodate up to ten quests. There was a pavilion that contained men's' and women's' dressing rooms, complete with showers and lockers, and cabinets containing various size swimsuits and cover-ups, and towels for use by guests. In between the dressing rooms was a sauna that could seat up to ten guests comfortably. Finally, there was an open-air bar well stocked with libations, both imported and domestic. Eighty-inch ultra-high-definition televisions with screens designed for outdoor viewing hung at both ends of the bar.

"Erik and Ksenia, welcome to our home," said Kristian. "Can I get you something to drink?"

"Thanks, Kristian," said Erik. "So great to be here with family and close friends. Happy Thanksgiving to everyone. What you're drinking looks interesting. Can I try one of those?"

"Certainly. Ksenia?"

"Yes, I would like the same."

"Help yourselves to the hors d'oeuvres," said Kristian. Several dishes, including small quiches, creamy garlic shrimp dip, crab leg pieces, sushi, and crab cakes, were spread out on one of the round redwood tables in front of the bar. "If you like, go find yourselves a swimsuit in the locker rooms and enjoy the pool and hot tub." So far, none of the guests took Kristian up on the offer as the November air was still quite cool, with temperatures in the low seventies.

Just then, the elevator door opened, and Miquel brought in another guest. Scarlett stepped out of the elevator, briefly waving to the group.

"Scarlett, do come in and join the party," said Ansley.

"Thanks for having me," said Scarlett. "You have a beautiful home. I was glad to receive your invitation. The thought of spending Thanksgiving in the Center alone was depressing."

Erik realized that all four of the cyborgs were present at a social gathering and was worried that their secret may be inadvertently revealed to Ksenia. Ksenia was the only adult present who did not know of the cyborg program. They would be together for several hours and Aaron had a tendency to speak before thinking. He had recently cautioned Scarlett before their dinner out the previous week that Ksenia did not know of the program. As soon as the opportunity arose, he would speak to both Kristian and Aaron discreetly. He saw Kristian was behind the bar preparing a couple of drinks and walked over.

"Kristian, I need to caution you that Ksenia does not know of the cyborg program. I haven't been able to get approval to let her in on it from the Navy. We need to exercise caution around her today."

"Understand. You two make a great couple. I hope you're able to resolve your... issue with the military soon. But when you do, Ansley would be happy to help Ksenia understand what it's like to be married to a cyborg. Also, Aaron and Savannah are getting serious. Maybe Ksenia could speak with Savannah as well."

"Thanks, Kristian. I've been genuinely concerned with how Ksenia will take the news when I'm able to reveal it to her. I will definitely suggest that she discuss any issues or concerns with Ansley and Savannah when the time comes."

Sitting at one table, Erik and Ksenia were joined by Scarlett, Savannah, and Aaron. "Scarlett, how is your rehab coming now that Erik has taken over your training?" asked Savannah.

"Quite well, actually. Erik pushes me to do a little more each day and I am feeling quite strong at this point. I hope to resume my aviation career soon."

"We need to continue to work on body coordination, hand-eye coordination so that you regain muscle memory lost with the amputations—memory that is immediately reactive and does not require thought before you jump in an airplane. But that will come soon," said Erik. "Once you are ready, I recommend extended time in the flight simulator before you do actual flying. In the meantime, we'll continue exercises that enhance development, as well as playing virtual reality video games that help create muscle memory."

Scarlett laughed. "I never thought I'd be training using video games, but they seem to help my ability to react quickly to various situations. The need to think about movement of my synthetic, er, artificial… limbs is becoming less each day." She detected Erik's stare at the near revelation of her actual condition.

At around 4:00 PM Miquel stepped out of the elevator and announced that dinner was ready and being served in the dining room on the first floor. The guests proceeded to the first floor and were seated at the long mahogany dining table. A large crystal candelabra chandelier hung over the table. Kristian stood at the head of the table and Ansley sat in the first chair to his right. Kristen Elaine sat in the first chair to his left. The table could accommodate up to 20 guests, so Ansley would be separated from the rest of the party had she sat in the traditional spot at the other end of the table, facing Kristian. The other guests sat on either side.

"Kristian, please give the blessing," said Ansley.

Kristian gave thanks for their home, each other and their daughter, their good health, and that of their guests. He also gave thanks for the country and for those that serve. Before him was a large roasted turkey, which he began carving and placing portions on plates that Ansley held and passed to the guests. They then passed around the sides, including mashed potatoes, dressing, several casseroles, and gravy. A butler dressed in a tuxedo with tails poured each guest's preference for white or red wine, brought directly from the mansion wine cellar.

Kristian then raised his glass in a toast. "May we all enjoy this day of thanksgiving and remember good times, good company, and good food."

"The food is exquisite," said Ksenia. "I like this Thanksgiving holiday."

"Thank you, Ksenia," said Ansley. "Do you have a similar holiday in Norway?"

"Norwegians do not celebrate a similar holiday. But we know of Thanksgiving as most Americans who are in Norway during the holiday celebrate."

As the main course finished, the butler and maid collected the dishes. In a few minutes, they returned with the traditional desserts including pumpkin, pecan and apple pies with whipped topping served in a sterling silver bowl.

"And these," pointing to the desserts, "are why Americans gain weight during the holidays. They look irresistible," said Aaron.

"I feel it is my duty to sample each of the desserts," said Erik, laughing.

After dinner, the men retired to a second-floor study next to Kristian's office, where Kristian poured cognac or brandy for his quests.

The ladies sat in the parlor, which was decorated in Nineteenth Century San Francisco-style furnishings, next to the dining room. The favorite after-dinner drink was the Vodka Cranberry Shrub or Vodka Cran, apple cider vinegar and fresh allspice berries joined with fresh cranberries in the shrub, along with some sugar to even out the flavor.

"Kristian hates this room," said Ansley. "says it reminds him of a brothel. When I asked him how he knew what a Nineteenth Century brothel looked like, he replied 'go watch Gone with the Wind, the scene at Belle Watling's place.'"

After a brief laugh by all the ladies, Ksenia said, "I think it is uniquely attractive. Sitting here gives one the sense of being sent back in time."

"Has anyone heard from the Guardian?" asked Kristian.

The others nodded negatively.

"Do we know if the Guardian has contacted Scarlett?" Aaron asked.

"Yes, he has," responded Erik. "Scarlett and I had a long conversation regarding the Guardian and what she should expect. She will be a great addition to our team."

"I think she has the hots for you, Erik," blurted out Aaron. "I could see the way she was looking at you dreamily at dinner."

Erik laughed and waved his hand to dismiss Aaron's comment. "Ksenia has my heart and soul."

Chapter Thirteen

Monday, December 1, 2042.

Scarlett texted Erik at 7:00 AM. "Did you get the email from Captain Barnes?"

Erik, still sleepy, rolled out of bed, picked up his smartphone and opened his email. Topping the list of messages was one from Captain Jeffrey Barnes, addressed to both Erik and Scarlett. "Please make yourselves available for a holographic conference call with SecDef at 1300 hours (1:00 PM) EST today. Dial-in information follows."

"1300 hours EST is in less than three hours! I hope I have a clean uniform ready," said Erik. He then returned Scarlett's text, confirming he had received the email from Barnes.

Ksenia, still groggy with sleep, rolled over and said, "Erik? Who are you talking to?"

"Myself. I have an important conference call with the Secretary of Defense in less than three hours."

While in the shower, he realized Barnes had not provided the topic or topics for discussion during the conference call. That stirred his imagination, wondering what SecDef would want with Scarlett and him. Several thoughts rushed through his mind, including the fate of the cyborg program, the status of the starship project, and Scarlett's rehab. Then he realized Scarlett may have contacted SecDef regarding his request to share the cyborg program with Ksenia. Did Scarlett really contact SecDef after he told her not to? This may not go well today.

Still dripping from his quick shower, he wrapped a towel around his waist and went back into the bedroom to get his smartphone. Replying to the email from Barnes, he typed "Topic for discussion?" and hit send. He continued to dry off and began dressing when he heard his phone buzz, indicating a new email had arrived.

"None provided. Guess we'll wait for the meeting."

Barnes' reply just made Erik more nervous. He texted Scarlett: "Can you meet me in the Center cafeteria at 0800?"

Scarlett replied, "Yes."

Sitting at a table away from others in the cafeteria, Erik said, "Do you have any idea why SecDef called this meeting today?"

"No, not really," said Scarlett, looking away.

"Scarlett, did you write to SecDef regarding my issue with telling Ksenia about my... condition?"

"Well, yes, I wrote to SecDef after we spoke. I referenced your situation in the letter to illustrate my concerns with the position he is taking."

"Great!" Erik said, his voice raising in anger. "So now we both get to look forward to an ass-chewing from the Secretary of Defense!"

"Hey, this is not only about you, Erik. I hope to have a serious relationship and wed in the future, and I don't feel the policy is fair."

At 12:45 PM Erik and Scarlett sat in a conference room that was configured for holographic communications. There was no small talk between them as both were not at all happy to be there expecting the meeting with SecDef and Captain Barnes. At 12:58 PM the holographic meeting equipment came alive, and Captain Barnes appeared to be seated across the table from Erik and Scarlett. At exactly 1300 hours (1:00 PM) Secretary of Defense William Bonner appeared to be seated next to Captain Barnes.

"Captain, Commander, Lieutenant, thank you for meeting with

me on short notice," said SecDef. "Lieutenant, I received your memo late last Wednesday. I understand your concerns and those of Commander Richards. I gave your memo some serious thought over the Thanksgiving holiday and have concluded that we, the U.S. military, need to do everything we can to support the health and wellbeing of those who choose to join the cyborg program. We will still strictly control with whom we share information regarding the cyborg program. So, I have spoken with the president and he has agreed to the following. Members of the program, specifically those who transition to a cyborg existence, will submit the name of anyone they wish to disclose their medical condition. Those who are submitted must be in a close relationship with the member. Candidates submitted for approval will undergo a thorough background investigation to ensure against unauthorized disclosure of the program by nefarious individuals who may compromise the program. Upon satisfactorily passing the background investigation, the candidate will be presented with the non-disclosure agreement associated with being accepted into the cyborg program. If the candidate agrees with the non-disclosure agreement and signs same, they will be eligible to receive information from the sponsoring member pertaining only to that member. Penalty for violating the agreement will be the same for a disclosure candidate as it is for a member and carries penalties akin to the crime of treason. Do you have questions?"

The room was silent for several seconds before Erik spoke. "So, in my case with Ksenia Anderson, I can submit her name as a disclosure candidate before I propose to her?"

"Yes, with the previously mentioned stipulations. Note that the background investigation will include at least one face-to-face interview with a senior military officer who may or may not be aware of the cyborg program, as well as a polygraph test."

After a few more seconds of silence, Scarlett said, "Mr. Secretary, I have no questions. Thank you, sir."

SecDef nodded at Scarlett's comment and said, "Captain Barnes, I am placing you in charge of a program to process requests for disclosure of the program to approved candidates. Please draft the policy and submit it to my attention as soon as possible. I believe the commander is urgently awaiting to hear next steps regarding his relationship." SecDef then left the meeting, his image fading, then disappearing from the room.

"Well, that was… interesting," said Captain Barnes. "You must have made quite a convincing case, Lieutenant. I wouldn't know because you bypassed the chain-of-command with your letter to SecDef. I hope you understand the seriousness of breaking the chain-of-command in the United States Navy. Ship captains have lost their command by breaking the chain-of-command."

"I am truly sorry, sir," said Scarlett. "It won't happen again."

"You realize I could put you in for an Article 32 hearing?"

"Yes, sir."

"Did Commander Richards put you up to this?" said Barnes, the sternness in his voice reflecting his lingering anger.

"No, sir," said Scarlett. "In fact, he asked me not to send a letter to SecDef."

"I will need to consider the events we have experienced today. In the meantime, you two draft the policy described by SecDef and have it on my desk by 0800 EST tomorrow morning. And if either of you break the chain-of-command again while I am your commanding officer, I'll see to it you spend the rest of your careers flying toilet paper to the ISS (International Space Station) after you get out of Leavenworth." Barnes' image then faded and disappeared as he left the meeting.

"I guess Barnes was pissed," said Scarlett.

"Ya think?!" said Erik.

"Well, it all worked out in the end, right?"

"I suppose I owe you thanks for sticking our necks out," said Erik.

Erik and Scarlett worked late into the evening, drafting the policy requested by SecDef. After several revisions and edits, they submitted the policy attached to an encrypted email to Captain Barnes. Erik also included a sample submission request naming

Ksenia as a candidate for disclosure of the cyborg program, hoping to speed along getting her approved.

Erik returned to the guest cottage about 9:00 PM. "Long day, hon?" said Ksenia.

"Yes, a very long day, but it was mostly good. I need to discuss something with you. But first, could you get me a beer?" said Erik as he sat on the teal sofa.

"Sure. What do you need to discuss with me?

"I have requested the Navy to allow me to disclose the… project I am working on to you. They have tentatively agreed, but you will be subjected to a background investigation before they give final approval."

"That doesn't sound like too big a deal," said Ksenia. "I had background checks when I was accepted to Kings Point, and when I applied to Viking."

"This one may be a little more intense. They will require you to take a lie-detector test, and you will be interviewed by a senior military officer."

"Wow, this project must be really important if they are going to spend that amount of time and money checking me out."

"That's not all. Before they will allow me to advise you regarding the project, you will need to sign a non-disclosure agreement that will prohibit you from disclosing the project to anyone else."

"O… K."

"The penalty for both purposeful and accidental disclosure to an unapproved party is the same as that for the crime of treason. I have signed the non-disclosure agreement."

"Oh, my… doesn't the crime of treason carry a death sentence?" asked Ksenia, concern reflected by her accent growing slightly stronger.

"A death sentence is not automatic or required, but it can be applied for treason."

"So, I could be sentenced to death for the slip of the tongue?" asked Ksenia, her Norwegian accent stronger yet. "I don't know. Perhaps I should just decline to know about your project."

"I understand your concern. I had concerns as well. But believe me when I tell you that you want to know about the project. It affects our future."

"Are you telling me that if I refuse to sign this agreement that you will break up with me?"

"No, that is definitely not what I am saying. But if you don't sign, it will prevent us from taking our relationship to the next step, which may ultimately result in us mutually agreeing to end the relationship. That would be tragic."

They sat in silence for several minutes. Then Ksenia said, "I love you, Erik, so I trust you. So, if you say that I need to sign this non-disclosure, I will sign it."

Erik said nothing but pulled her close to him where they remained for quite a while.

Chapter Fourteen

Kristian had just attached his charging/backup cable to the back of his neck and lay down. As he drifted into his mind's resting state, a mist began forming at the end of his bed. The mist formed into a familiar shape and The Guardian materialized out of the mist. The Guardian summoned Kristian's spirit. His synthetic body remained on the bed next to Ansley, who was fast asleep.

"Kristian, please grab my arm. We will raise the others. We have serious work to do. A timeline is threatening your existence and that of billions."

Kristian did as he was told and was instantly transported to Erik's bedside. Erik's spirit arose and departed his synthetic body while Ksenia slept. The three then appeared to Scarlett and Aaron, and all were led by The Guardian to an unknown place in the year 2028. Once the assignment was completed, all four were returned to the exact moment in time they were arisen by The Guardian.

"I will now show you why we have come here. The year is 2028 and we are in China near the province of Wuhan. You may recall that a virology laboratory in Wuhan was found to be the source of the SARS Covid-II Virus that devastated the world in 2020. Although the Chinese government vigorously denied it, many thought the virus was a bioweapon manufactured by the Chinese military. The reality is the Chinese were indeed developing a bioweapon, but the still experimental SARS Covid II virus escaped the lab because of negligence.

"The continued development of the virus bioweapon is a creation wholly sponsored by the Chinese military. A coronavirus that is the basis for the common cold and the SARs viruses is weaponized with a warhead that can infect all human beings and for which there is no natural immunity, antidote, vaccine, or cure. After the pandemic of 2020-2021, the Chinese continued to develop the bioweapon into a much deadlier pathogen that can cause rapid death in targeted segments of the global population. Using DNA markers specific to a targeted race, its payload causes symptoms like those resulting from nerve gas weapons in the targeted race while leaving other races asymptomatic. The latest iteration of the virus targets the Caucasian race. The virus causes intense sweating, filling of the bronchial passages with mucus, dimming of vision, uncontrollable vomiting and defecation, convulsions, and finally paralysis and respiratory failure. Death results from asphyxia within hours of exposure. The goal of the Chinese Communist Party (CCP) is to exterminate the population of most of North America and Europe to make room for the expanding Asian race, now numbering close to two billion, and to eliminate the greatest resistance to global domination.

"I will now show you the outcome should this deadly virus be deployed."

The four cyborgs watched in silence as images of people dying with excruciating symptoms flowed before their minds' eye. Images of major cities in Europe and North America showed masses of people dying in the streets, in office buildings, in vehicles, and in private homes. Caucasian emergency and medical personnel were of no use as they, too, were dying quickly. Non-Caucasian emergency personnel, doctors, nurses and EMTs were quickly overwhelmed with the number of people seeking treatment for the virus which had no antidote or cure. People of mixed-race backgrounds also fell to the pathogen if they had Caucasian DNA, which left only approximately ten percent of the population of North America and six percent of the population of Europe to survive. Earth-moving machines and bulldozers, driven by non-Whites, were seen digging massive trenches and moving mounds of bodies into them. Many religious leaders were claiming the End of Times was upon them, while others claimed God was punishing the evil ways man had adopted. The population of Earth was reduced from nine billion to three billion in a matter of weeks. Following these images, images revealed the Chinese army marching on capital cities and the flag of the People's Republic of China flying over Paris, London, Washington, D.C., Ottawa, Bonn, Rome, and other major cities.

"We will now travel inside the Wuhan CCP laboratory, where fifty political prisoners have been assembled for experimentation using the deadly virus. The group comprises ten Caucasians, ten Blacks, ten Asians, ten Australoid, and ten of mixed race that possess markers of Caucasian DNA."

The four cyborg spirits then found themselves with The Guardian in what appeared to be a control room. Technicians in full anti-contamination suits appeared to be preparing for a test. In their spirit form, the cyborgs understood any human language perfectly. They faced a wall with a large window looking in on the fifty test subjects, all dressed in gray jumpsuits, milling about the room. One technician appeared to be the lead and began issuing orders to the others.

"Have we received the reports for labs taken from each of the subjects this morning?" asked the lead technician.

"We have. All the subjects appear to be in excellent health."

To get test results closely emulating real-world conditions, the test subjects who were political prisoners of the CCP had been restored to good health. Previously, most were in poor physical condition, depending on the length of their time in prison, where they were given only enough nutrients to keep them alive. The selection process eliminated any candidate test subjects if they were suffering from any disease. Until today, all the test subjects were enjoying the benefits of bountiful, healthful nutrition for the past several months to prepare for the test about to be conducted.

"Verify and acknowledge that your anti-contamination suit and breathing apparatus works properly," said the lead.

All the technicians responded affirmatively.

"Release the virus!" exclaimed the lead.

A technician touched an icon on a video display and a large test tube appeared on the displays in the control room. The contents of the test tube slowly diminished until the tube was empty, showing the virus had been deployed.

At first, none of the test subjects exhibited any reaction as the invisible virus permeated the test room. Then, approximately forty minutes after the virus was released, a few of the Caucasian and two of the mixed-race subjects appeared to be sweating. After another twenty minutes had passed, all the Caucasian subjects and the two of mixed race that had originally exhibited symptoms were exhibiting more severe symptoms, including sweating, nausea and vomiting, and foaming at the mouth. The remaining eight mixed-race subjects began exhibiting some symptoms, including sweating and nausea. None of the other subjects exhibited symptoms but watched, horrified, as their Caucasian and mixed-race colleagues fell to the floor in convulsions. In a little over an hour, all twenty subjects having Caucasian DNA markers were dead.

"Guardian, we must stop this!" exclaimed Kristian.

"Unfortunately, we cannot stop the cruelty you are witnessing today. But we have a plan to save humanity," replied the Guardian without emotion. Noting the four cameras mounted near the ceiling of the test room, he continued, "This event today was recorded. One technician present here today will be so overwhelmed by the effects of the virus that she can be… persuaded to copy the recording and escape to the United States. We will visit her in a dream and… suggest that she do so and provide her with a plan to execute this action. Since she is a woman, Scarlett will be tasked with fulfilling this assignment."

After all the subjects that had fallen had been verified as

deceased, the other subjects were escorted from the room. Most were shaken, some had tears rolling down their cheeks, while others were weeping. All showed signs of fear.

The leader then declared the test complete.

Chapter Fifteen

"Scarlett, Li Jing is the name of the laboratory technician we saw being repulsed by the results of the virus test. She will be the first target of our intervention in preventing the release of the virus by the Chinese Communist military. Tonight, you will enter Li Jing's mind as a vivid dream and plant the suggestion to capture a copy of the video of today's experiment and get it into the hands of the United States Central Intelligence Agency. Along with the… suggestion, you will provide Li with instructions on how to hack into the Wuhan lab's video library and download the video to her smartphone. Once downloaded, she will transmit the encrypted video to an address in the CIA's electronic vault."

"Sounds good, Guardian, but how will Li Jing's transmission of the video go undetected by the CCP?" asked Adam. "I'm sure the CCP has tight reins on what gets transmitted out of this lab, especially to an address outside of China."

"This will require coordination on our part. Still under observation by Scarlett, when Li Jing touches the 'send' icon on her smartphone, Scarlett will notify Erik, who is standing by in the lab's communication control room. Erik will then enter the mind of the technician on duty to monitor communications. Erik will block the technician from seeing the visual and hearing the audible alarms associated with an unapproved transmission. The initial address of the CIA to which the transmission is sent will employ a VPN within China. This will reduce concern should an audit reveal the transmission."

"Kristian's role will be to monitor the analyst observing communications traffic for the CIA. Kristian will force the analyst to view the contents of the video file. However, the analyst will probably open the file without Kristian's influence because of her own curiosity. Once the analyst has viewed the file, we expect she will forward it to the proper staff within the CIA who will bring the video to the CIA director and ultimately to the Joint Chiefs and the president. We will monitor all activity and intervene as needed to see the proper delivery and outcome of the video."

Chapter Sixteen

The plan for the capture and delivery of the video of the gruesome experiment at the Wuhan Laboratory went off with only a minor hitch. The Chinese technician monitoring communications sent from the lab's location noticed the transmission sent from Li Jing's smart phone when he saw and heard the alarms showing an unapproved transmission had been sent. But Erik quickly entered and got control of the technician and controlled his senses of hearing and vision, so he only saw the alarm for less than one second. The technician, who felt something strange when Erik entered his mind, concluded the warnings to be false alarms.

At CIA headquarters in Langley, Virginia, several senior analysts viewed the video. The audio portion was translated from Mandarin to English by an auto-translator. The conclusion of the analysts was that the Chinese were indeed conducting experiments using pathogens on different races with the apparent targeting of Caucasians. Some were briefly confused when the video showed those appearing to be of mixed race also were affected. But others correctly surmised that the mixed-race individuals also had Caucasian DNA markers. After several days of analysis, including that of the video itself to ensure its authenticity, the senior analyst group recommended that the video be shown to the Director.

A meeting was setup with the Director, Mark Hamilton, and three of the most senior analysts who had reviewed the video. Also included in the meeting were the Assistant Director of Covert Operations, Allan Quinn, and the Assistant Director of Agency Communications, Marie Samuels. Director Hamilton opened the meeting.

"I understand that you gentlemen and lady have something you have deemed of great importance to national security to show us this morning," said Director Hamilton.

"Sir, we believe the Communist Chinese Military, under the direction of the CCP, is planning to release another pandemic. Further, we believe this weapon will target those with Caucasian DNA markers while leaving the remaining races on the planet unscathed." The lead analyst then touched an icon on the screen in front of him embedded in the table. The video then played and revealed a timestamp at the bottom of the screen to enable fast-forwarding, rewind, and pause.

At the conclusion of the video, the room was silent for what seemed like several minutes, but was less than one minute. "Has this video been validated for authenticity, Marie?" said Director Hamilton.

"Unfortunately, yes, it has," replied Samuels.

"And how did you conclude that this virus will selectively attack people of a specific race?" questioned Hamilton.

"Sir, if you watch the video closely, you see that only those who appear to be Caucasian and perhaps those who have some Caucasian features are affected by the virus. Shall I replay the video for you, sir?"

"No, I noticed what you have observed. Do we have any traffic coming out of China that shows the release of the virus is imminent?"

"No traffic of that nature has been intercepted, Director," said Marie Samuels. "But recall that the Chinese withheld information regarding the release of the SARS-CoV-2 virus in 2019 effectively, and then lied to the world regarding its potential effects."

"I will request time with the President, the Secretary of State, and Joint Chiefs to review what we have here," said Hamilton. "The CIA will not be held responsible for burying what could be an existential threat to not only the United States, but to much of the world's population."

The Guardian then turned to face the four spirits who took part in the mission to expose the CCP's plan to eradicate much of the world's population. "I will now return you to the moment I awoke you for this mission. I will watch the development of the response to the video we saw delivered to a member of the president's cabinet. When actions on your part are called for, I will engage you all."

With that, the four cyborg spirits each found themselves back in their beds, awake but somewhat stunned at what had just transpired.

Chapter Seventeen

rik lay in bed next to Ksenia, wide awake after his latest adventure with The Guardian. He thought, "We went back in time to 2028. By virtue of the fact that I am laying here in 2042, unscathed and unchanged, shows the overall mission to thwart China in its plans to release the deadly pathogen was successful. I don't recall any of this being in the press, which shows the entire event was kept from the public across multiple countries. I will need to do some research on this starting tomorrow morning."

Erik never could put his mind into its full resting state before light could be seen between the slats in the window shades. Thoughts of the mission with The Guardian and thinking about Ksenia's invitation to join her in Norway for Christmas and proposing to Ksenia were competing in his mind for attention. Looking at the clock next to the bed, he saw it was 0642. Ksenia was still sound asleep when he slipped out of bed, grabbed his robe, and went into the kitchen to make coffee.

He made coffee, with cream and sugar, and sat down with his smartphone in the great room. He saw he had received an email from Captain Barnes at 0406 local time, which would have been 0706 on the East Coast. Thinking that the email must be important for the captain to send it the day after Thanksgiving, the email read "Request for leave 17 Dec-05 Jan approved. Please fwd plans for Groom Lake next week."

"Oh, shit!" thought Erik. "I almost forgot about the trip to Area 51. With the holiday weekend, I will need to scramble to get the itinerary ready and sent to the attendees."

Just then, Ksenia walked from the bedroom to the kitchen to pour coffee. "Good morning, love," she said, smiling. "You're up early this morning."

"Yes, I had several things on my mind that I needed to attend to. Captain Barnes approved my leave for our Norway trip."

"Wonderful," said Ksenia, joining Erik on the sofa after pouring her coffee. "I know you're going to love Norway at Christmas. We have many traditions you will find… interesting when compared with your American Christmas."

"Are you sure that your parents want me to stay for over two weeks?"

"They will be thrilled to hear that you can stay throughout the holidays. Even Thor said he is looking forward to OUR return."

"You mean Thor is looking forward to your return?"

"He used the words '… looking forward to your and Erik's visit…' in his text message. Would you like to see it?"

"No, I trust you, I think," said Erik, grinning at her.

"What do you mean, you think?" bristled Ksenia, grabbing a pillow to throw at Erik.

The pillow fight escalated to foreplay and ended with a quick bout of lovemaking on the sofa. "OK, I trust you," said Erik, now on top of and nose -to-nose with Ksenia.

"Where's my pillow? I'm gonna beat you again!" yelled Ksenia.

Chapter Eighteen

The day after Thanksgiving, 2042. Immediately after Erik had provided Captain Barnes with the meeting itinerary for Groom Lake just before noon PST, Barnes returned with the following message. "Please include Lt. Bross in your plans for Groom Lake. Now that she has transitioned, she can join your team. I will send her orders."

Erik realized he hadn't previously considered Scarlett for the starship team, but understood where Barnes was going with this. A crew comprising as many cyborgs as possible was necessary since the leading technology supporting suspended animation for long-duration space travel had not been successfully tested. He also knew there had been a discussion of transitioning healthy non-cyborg crew members to synthetic bodies. Even at the speed of light, a trip to the nearest habitable planet would take years, even decades. Also, dealing with human body illnesses on a trip of that length could be very distracting.

Scarlett heard the tone showing she had received an encrypted, secure email message from SPACECOM. Opening the message, which required she hold the camera of her smartphone in front of her eyes, she saw the official stamp showing that the message contained orders. She read the email which stated that she was officially assigned to a top-secret project and to report immediately to Commander Erik Richards for details.

Erik heard his smartphone ping, showing an incoming video message. He saw the message was from Scarlett, so he put the phone into holographic display mode. A 3-D image of Scarlett was broadcast from his smartphone. "LT. Scarlett Bross reporting for duty, sir," she said. "SPACECOM just assigned me to a project you're heading up. Care to provide the details?"

"Let's meet for lunch at 1300 in the cafeteria and I will bring you up to speed. In the meantime, start packing. We're leaving on a trip on Monday for three days. Destination is Groom Lake, Nevada."

The cafeteria at Barnett Center was open the day after Thanksgiving, but only for items available from its vending machines. Erik grabbed a tuna salad sandwich and a coke and sat at a table in the back of the large room. Scarlett soon entered the cafeteria and got a chef salad out of the vending machine, along with a bottle of water. She saw Erik at the back of the cafeteria and noted that there were only a few people in the room, all out of hearing range from Erik's table.

As Scarlett sat down, Erik commented, "you know you are no longer restricted to a diet of bunny food, right?"

"Old habits are hard to break," said Scarlett, followed by a brief laugh. "So, what is this top-secret project that I've been shanghaied for? Did you get me assigned to it?"

"The United States is developing humanity's first starship. SPACECOM is partnering with several close allies and the private sector on building a spacecraft capable of deep space exploration. Much of the ship's design has been gained through efforts that began as early as the 1950s to discover the design and engineering behind an alien spacecraft that crashed in 1947 in Arizona."

Scarlett just stared at Erik for nearly thirty seconds. "To my knowledge, I do not believe we've ever solved the mystery behind the UFO sightings around naval vessels first revealed to the public around 2020. I actually saw one of these things when flying off the

USS Ronald Reagan in the Atlantic shortly after getting my wings. It was there, visually and on my radar, one moment, then gone the next. My cameras recorded it, so I wasn't hallucinating. When I landed, the chips were immediately removed from my cameras by ship security personnel. I heard nothing more about the incident."

"There's a lot more to the story, Scarlett," said Erik, still chewing his first bite of his sandwich. Swallowing, he continued, "Many of the stories around Area 51 and the crash of a UFO are actually true. You will see things that will literally shock you when we tour Area 51 next week. Not only did a real spacecraft crash in 1947, it had a crew. Unfortunately, those occupants that did not perish in the crash could not be revived. But what we know now is that the occupants were cyborgs–part biological, part machine. Like you and me, their bodies were apparently controlled by minds from biological bodies that were harvested and downloaded to the synthetic bodies. The energy sources that enabled the cyborgs were millions of nano-sized batteries embedded in their skin. The batteries were charged using ambient light, so there was no need to plug in for periodic charging. I understand that Ansley's team is developing a similar battery array for synthetic bodies like ours. Of course, in 1947 we had no knowledge of the physiology or design of the alien synthetic bodies, so the one alien cyborg still alive after the crash could not be revived. It never regained consciousness and eventually 'died' after its nano-batteries were exhausted. Apparently, had we known more, all we may have had to do was expose the body to sunlight and its batteries may have recharged. But it was kept in a body bag for several days while it was shipped to Wright-Patterson. Even then, had we known that all it needed was a sunbath, we may have been able to revive it. But we didn't understand the means of recharging the body until recently. That is why you and I have more conventional, bulkier batteries located where our kidneys would be in a human body."

"Where are these alien bodies now?" asked Scarlett.

"The one that survived but later perished was sent back to Area 51 for storage when it became apparent that we could not revive it at Wright-Pat. The other three are also kept in storage at Area 51. You will see the bodies next week."

"What do they look like? Us?"

"They aren't dissimilar to us. Large skull, two large eyes, mouth, four limbs, bipedal. They are taller and thinner than we are, which may result from a lower gravity on their home planet."

"So, intelligent life elsewhere in the Universe is true. Do we have any idea where these beings came from?"

"It is my understanding that the navigation systems on the ship that crashed in 1947 have finally been understood. Twelve light years from Earth is the star system that appears to be the origin of the craft. The star in question is Tau Ceti and is visible to the naked eye. The planets surrounding the star are estimated to be two to six times bigger than earth, with one measuring five times the size of our home planet. Said planet is lying in what's commonly known as the star's 'Goldilocks Zone'—a position that is neither too hot nor too cold, but exactly the right environment to support the prospect of liquid surface water, and therefore, life. Assuming that the alien craft can achieve near-light speed, twelve years is a reasonable length of time for a synthetic being to travel."

"If that planet is five times the size of Earth, it would have significantly greater gravity than Earth. How do you explain your idea that the height of the aliens could be due to lower gravity in their home world?"

"Don't forget, we are not seeing the bodies of an actual corporeal being from that world. We have been transmitting video and audio out into space for over one hundred years. It is possible the synthetic bodies of the crew were designed for Earth's gravity and to look as much like us as possible. Again, given the technology necessary to travel twelve light years across the galaxy, anything is possible."

"Our synthetic bodies aren't designed for a constant five G's are they?" asked Scarlett.

"They may be. Look at the strength that we have compared to normal humans," said Erik. "We have a wheels-up time of 0700 on Monday morning. It will be an excellent opportunity to see how well your new body can handle a T-38. I'll be your WSO (Weapons Systems Officer–back seat)."

"You think I'm ready for that?" said Scarlett, with a surprised look on her face.

"You've done pretty well in the simulator. Time to get back in the saddle, Lieutenant. Oh, Ksenia and I are hosting a barbeque on Sunday. Why don't you plan on joining us? Festivities will start about 1300."

"Thanks. I'll plan on it."

Chapter Nineteen

Monday after Thanksgiving, 2042, 7:00 AM. Scarlett (call sign Tara) is at the controls of a T-38 Talon sitting on Runway 27 at Los Angeles Air Force Base (LAAFB) awaiting instructions for takeoff. Erik is in the backseat.

"Tara, you're cleared for takeoff. At three zero (3,000) feet, set your heading to zero-three-zero."

"Rolling, Tara. Have a good day," said Scarlett as the T-38 began its takeoff roll, climbed to three thousand feet and banked right to a heading of zero-three-zero degrees, bound for Groom Lake, Nevada. "Great to be back on the flight deck," said Scarlett. "I have missed this. Care for a barrel roll, Erik?"

"Go for it, pilot," said Erik, as Scarlett put the T-38 into a tight roll.

Forty-five minutes after departure from Los Angeles: "Tara, Homey Approach Control. Clear to land, Runway 13R, wind two-one-zero at fourteen."

"Homey Tower, clear to land Runway 13R, Tara," said Scarlett.

After landing the T-38, Scarlett was instructed to taxi to an unidentified hangar at the end of the ramp where a black SUV was parked. As they came to a stop, the driver and an additional armed man stepped out of the vehicle and stood at the door.

"Good afternoon, Commander Richards, Lieutenant Bross. Commander, good to see you again. Lieutenant, I am Captain Sean Miller, U.S. Air Force. With me is Staff Sergeant James. We will take you to meet with our base commander, Colonel Jacobsen. The rest of your project team arrived last night and will meet us in the briefing."

"Commander Richards, good to see you again," said Colonel Jacobson. "You must be Lt. Bross," Jacobsen said to Scarlett, extending his hand to shake hers.

"Yes, sir. Nice to meet you," said Scarlett.

"Commander, your project team is right next door. Shall we join them?"

"Yes, sir," replied Erik.

As they entered the base briefing room, Colonel Jacobson said, "Some of us have already met, but let's go around the room and introduce ourselves. Commander?"

"I'll introduce my team," said Erik. Going clockwise around the table, Erik began, "To my right is Project System Engineering Manager Rick Williams, Deputy Project System Engineering Manager Kirk Banner, Chief Engineer Allan Stanner from Scotland, Deputy Chief Engineer Keith Callahan from Ireland, Deputy Chief Engineer Soren Amakov from Sweden, Flight Systems Manager Raymond Billings, and Chief Pilot candidate Lieutenant Scarlett Bross. This team was established over the past six months and represents the best aerospace project team in the world."

"Thank you, Commander," said Jacobson. "I believe you all have met Captain Miller, who will be your guide for your visit here. Captain, please begin the video and slide show for our guests."

A one-hundred-twenty-inch clear screen was lowered from the ceiling. Standing in front of the screen, Captain Miller clicked through a series of photographs of Area 51 and described the purpose of the facilities shown in each, just as he had done for Erik and Captain Barnes six months prior. Near the end of the briefing, the audience was shown the side of a mountain close to the base. This picture was actually a video that showed a large section of the mountainside fade away and reveal what appeared to be large hangar doors. The doors opened, and the camera zoomed inside the facility to reveal an oblong, windowless craft that resembled a dirigible in shape. It appeared to be floating a few feet above the floor.

"What you are seeing, gentlemen, is the craft that crash-landed near Roswell, New Mexico in 1947," said Colonel Jacobsen. "The United States has denied the existence of this craft for nearly one-hundred years and continues to deny it exists today. Approximately seventy years during this period have been spent trying to figure out how it works—what it's made of, its method of propulsion, and who built it. In the early 2020s, we were finally able to determine these things and reverse-engineer some of its components and systems. But much earlier, beginning in the 1950s, we were able to incorporate some of its basic designs into aircraft like the A-12, the SR-71 Blackbird, and later into the B-2 Bomber. During those years, we were decades ahead of any other country regarding stealth aircraft design. The large hangar facilities behind the illusionary mountainside were created with the help of high-powered laser cannons. The mountainside illusion covering the hangar doors is an ultra-high-resolution video beamed from hidden transmitters on the mountain. Part of the protected airspace surrounding the base is above the mountain. Aircraft that violate that airspace are warned that they are subject to being shot down should they enter the protected airspace. If they persist, laser cannons hidden on the mountain will fire and destroy the aircraft instantly by literally reducing it to atoms. There are no remnants of the aircraft nor human remains. The video transmitters on the mountain also block all visibility from space. Questions?"

The attendees sat speechless for what seemed like minutes after Captain Miller finished his presentation. Then, Chief Engineer Allan Stanner said in his noticeable Scottish accent, "How much have we learned about the spacecraft? Do we understand how the thing flew? What material is the hull made of? Do we know where the thing came from?"

"All questions that we will answer over the next couple of days as we tour the facility and examine the spacecraft," said Captain Miller. "Let's all head to the officers' club where lunch will be served."

As the group exited the officers' club after lunch, two plain black SUVs were waiting. Colonel Jacobson took the wheel of the leading vehicle and Captain Miller got into the driver's seat in the second. The two vehicles shared a private radio frequency so all the visitors could hear Jacobsen and Miller describe what they would see, and not see, on their way to the top-secret facility in the desert. Erik was the only person in the group who had seen the facility and its contents previously.

As they approached a mountain, its face dissolved slowly, revealing the one-hundred-foot-tall hangar doors. The doors opened just enough for the SUVs to enter the hangar. Just inside the hangar, an SR-71 Blackbird spy plane could be seen. The hangar doors closed immediately. Once closed, the image of the SR-71 dissolved, revealing the alien spacecraft they had seen the day before in the video. There were also armed guards wearing camouflage fatigues and carrying combat weapons posted on either side of the spacecraft. There was maximum security around the spacecraft and within the hangar.

The alien spacecraft was oval, wider towards the center than at the front and rear, tapering on the edges to a flat, narrow wing that appeared to be about one-meter wide that surrounded the craft. The craft measured twenty-two meters long, sixteen meters high, and sixteen meters wide at the center. There were no windows or hatches visible from outside the ship. The material used for the external skin appeared to be aluminum but seemed to adjust, as if alive. The craft floated about four feet above the hangar floor.

The group exited the two vehicles and followed Captain Miller walking towards the alien spacecraft. "There doesn't seem to be anything supporting that craft," said Chief Engineer Stanner. "How is it just floating in the air?"

"The craft uses anti-gravity technology for propulsion, which also allows it to hover at virtually any altitude. This technology also allows it to move at incredibly high rates of speed without a visible means of propulsion," said Miller.

"We believe the ship to be from a much larger spacecraft, similar in concept to our aircraft carriers," Miller continued. "Similar craft have been seen and filmed by military jets on several occasions beginning early in this century. Before that, we believe their stealth capabilities coupled with their incredible acceleration effectively hid them from our most advanced camera technologies."

"We believe the craft is capable of trans-atmospheric flight, enabling the craft to leave Earth's atmosphere. It is equipped with cabin-pressurization, inertial dampening, and life-support systems that are sophisticated enough to allow up to four crew members to sit comfortably inside the craft without requiring the need of sealed and pressurized space or G-suits, despite the craft's perceived ability to pull incredible-G turns that stress normal air-frames and pilots often to the breaking point. It is apparent, by the near-perfect condition of this ship, that the craft can complete re-entry into a planet's atmosphere at least as dense as Earth's."

"When this craft was found, it was embedded in a crater some forty feet deep. Much of the forward hull was crushed, including the flight deck. After it was excavated from the crater under the cover of strict military security, it was taken to Wright-Patterson Airforce Base in Ohio. Then it was brought to Area 51 when the first hangar was retrofitted with advanced, state-of-the-art security systems."

"After a few days, it became apparent that the craft was... healing itself. After about a month, there was no evidence that the craft had been nearly destroyed in the crash. We still don't know how that happened, but know that the material in the exterior hull is nothing like we have here on Earth."

"What happened to the crew?" asked Kirk Banner.

"Despite many rumors regarding the condition of the crew, two actually survived for a time. What we found appeared to be biological remains, but they were anything but. All four, we later determined, were completely synthetic."

"If you gentlemen will follow me, let's get on board." The party climbed a ladder and entered what appeared to be the flight deck of the alien craft. Captain Miller stepped forward, between two rows of two seats each, and waved his hand over a dial on the cockpit display panel. The forward section of the hull appeared to dissolve, revealing a completely clear, floor-to-ceiling view of the hangar doors in front of the craft. On the armrests of the two forward seats were joysticks, like those in a fly-by-wire jet aircraft that appeared to be for navigation and weapons control. Multiple screens could be seen on the cockpit display panel, but were all dark until Miller placed his hand on one of the forward seat armrests. Then the screens came alive, displaying what appeared to be the status of different systems on the ship, but with characters heretofore never seen by any of the team except Erik.

"The size and shape of the seats show they were for beings similar to humans," said Erik. "I believe you will be astounded at how much the alien cyborgs resemble humans."

"The little green men and other movie portrayals of alien beings were mostly figments of active imaginations," said Miller. "Not much else to show you, but if you follow me, we'll have a look at the aliens."

"Will we see how this ship operates? My engineers and I would sure like a peek at the propulsion and navigation systems before we leave. A look under the hood and kick the tires, so to speak."

"Yes, we have set aside most of the day tomorrow for your team to work with our engineers and learn as much as we know about the functioning of this craft," said Miller.

The project team entered a stark, white hallway that had no visible doors as far as they could see. Miller walked about thirty feet when he turned to face the right wall. A portal opened into a large room housing a long, oval conference table and chairs. Once they were inside, the opaque far wall dissolved into clear glass, revealing four metal operating tables. On each table there was a body. The bodies appeared to be hairless from head to foot. Feet were narrow and legs were long. The arms and hands were also thin. What appeared to be male reproductive organs were visible in the groin area of the torso, which was very human-like. The hands had four long fingers, and the feet had four large toes each. The hands and feet appeared proportionally larger than human hands and feet. The head appeared to be elongated with a high, wide forehead and very narrow chin. Eyes were larger than human eyes, rounded and tapered that gave the being an Asian-like appearance. The nose was long and narrow and appeared to have only one nostril. The mouth was small but very human-like, but there were no apparent lips.

"How have you kept them so well preserved for over ninety years?" asked Soren Amakov. "There is no apparent decay of their flesh."

"What you are seeing are not bodies of biological beings," continued Miller. "These bodies are artificial, synthetic. Near as we can determine, they are specifically designed for long space travel. The materials used are a combination of known synthetics that have compatible Earth material, and of initially unknown synthetics that took years for us to determine their atomic structure."

The tour of Area 51 continued through the following day into Wednesday. Engineering chief Stanner and his two deputy engineers, Systems Engineering Manager, Rick Williams Systems Engineering Manager and his deputy, Kirk Banner, spent the entire day Tuesday with the Area 51 engineers, combing the structure systems onboard the alien spacecraft. On Wednesday, the team members departed after a debriefing session with Erik and Captain Miller, and a tour of the new project headquarters that was under construction.

"Thank you for joining our tour this week, gentlemen," said Erik at the conclusion of the briefing. "I hope you have a most enjoyable and Merry Christmas. I will see you again at the Pentagon in January. Colonel Jacobson, Captain Miller, thank you for your hospitality and a most informative tour. Merry Christmas."

Chapter Twenty

As Erik and Scarlett flew from Groom Lake back to Los Angeles, Scarlett said, "That alien craft looked remarkably similar to the craft I saw when flying off of the Ronald Reagan. Do you know if the Air Force has flown this craft or one that is of similar design?"

"I've heard several rumors regarding an advanced Navy SPACECOM deployment in outer space, but I saw no evidence of its existence on my Mars trips," replied Erik. "I have heard the term 'Solar Warden' mentioned with this group. Rumors say that Solar Warden was charged with protecting Earth from attack by extraterrestrials, but I do not believe the group ever existed. However, I wouldn't discount the possibility that the Air Force is flight testing this or similar craft. There have been dozens of UFO sightings in this region over the past several decades."

Erik walked through the door of the guest cottage at Barnett Center about 4 PM. "Ksenia, I'm back," he said just as Ksenia came into the living room.

After they embraced, Ksenia said smiling, "How was your trip? Did you accomplish your mission?"

"Yes, I believe so. I'll need to write a mission report for Captain Barnes first thing in the morning."

"I tried to call Scarlett to see if she wanted to go out for lunch. Her virtual assistant said she was away, returning today. Did she go with you?"

"Yes, she was assigned to the project team by Captain Barnes."

Ksenia drew quiet for a moment and Erik, still holding her, could feel her tension rise. "I had nothing to do with her assignment to the team. It was Captain Barnes' order, and the trip was all business. Scarlett is a business colleague, nothing more," said Erik, gently, to erase the frown he could see forming on Ksenia's face.

Moving a step away from Erik, Ksenia said, "I hope that is all it is."

"Hey, you have nothing to be jealous over. Let's go out to the lanai and have a drink. It's nearly happy hour."

"I'm not jealous," she said, still pouting.

Nothing more was said by either Ksenia or Erik regarding Scarlett's appointment to Erik's project. But it wouldn't be the last time Scarlett's presence around Erik angered Ksenia. Ksenia's mood quickly lightened with the help of one of Erik's daiquiris. Drinks were followed by dinner, which was grilled hamburgers and French fries. As the light faded and the weather cooled, they moved inside. Erik lit a fire which led to lovemaking on a blanket on the floor in front of the fireplace and then later continued in the bedroom. While laying on the floor, after Ksenia had dosed off, Erik noticed the glow of the embers on her skin. He realized at that moment that he must not let this beauty ever leave him and kissed her.

Chapter Twenty-one

Erik arose early on Thursday and began writing his mission report on the trip to Area 51 when he paused, recalling the most recent engagement with The Guardian. He abandoned the report temporarily to research what the cyborg spirits had seen at the Chinese Virology Lab in Wuhan. First, he found a Newsmax article from 2021 where a journalist named Gordon Chang, who was very familiar with the Chinese Communist Party and President XI, was quoted. "(President) Xi knows he has spread" COVID-19 to the rest of the world, killing millions of people and that he can spread the next disease "with impunity, and we know the Chinese military researchers are working on pathogens they call specific ethnic genetic attacks." Apparently, Chang was eerily accurate as the article continued, "They will leave the Chinese immune and they will sicken and kill everybody else, which means the next disease from China could be a civilization killer, so there may very well be no America afterward."

He found only a few references to the lab that stated that the lab was destroyed in late 2028. Unconfirmed reports stated the lab was obliterated, flattened by what appeared to be lightning bolts that came from the sky. Erik knew the lab had been ground zero for the infamous Sars-1 and Sars-2 viruses, but saw no references to this in his internet searches. The lab was not only physically destroyed, but all references to its history had been removed from public access.

Erik next searched for a reaction by the Chinese to the lab's destruction and found that China had issued press releases indicating the lab had been destroyed by natural forces. Unable to find any concrete cause for the lab's destruction, he suspected some sort of coverup. This then sent his imagination spinning about the rumors he had heard about Solar Warden. Had the information on the deadly SARS-3 virus that the cyborg spirits guided to the Director of the CIA and ultimately to the President resulted in an attack on the lab? A conventional attack by the U.S., with or without its allies, on the lab would have resulted in a swift military response from the Chinese. That the lab was never rebuilt by the Chinese was also a curiosity. Coupled with the numerous sightings of unidentified aircraft near naval warships that continue to this day, many resembling the spacecraft Erik had seen at Area 51, further piqued his curiosity regarding a space-based attack. He concluded he would raise these questions with Captain Barnes when they met upon his return to The Pentagon in January.

Erik then returned to his report for Captain Barnes just as Ksenia walked into the living room. "Good morning, Erik, been up long?" she said, as she bent over his shoulder and kissed him on the cheek.

"Just finishing up my report on the trip to Nevada for Captain Barnes," he said. "Coffee is ready."

"Have you made reservations for our trip to Norway? It's coming up quickly."

"I will do that as soon as I finish the report, in just a few minutes," he replied without looking up from the laptop screen.

"Ksenia, when and where do you need to pick up your next ship assignment in January?" asked Erik.

"My cruise leaves on January third, so I need to be in Miami on January second. Which means we will need to leave my parent's home and drive to Bergen on New Year's Day."

"OK, I will book us both to Miami. I don't report back to the

Pentagon until January fifth. Do you have a hotel preference in Miami?"

"The Hyatt Regency near the port is nice."

Erik then booked their flights to Bergen on December 17, 2042, with return to Miami on January 2, 2043. He also booked a suite at the Hyatt Regency near the Port of Miami.

Chapter Twenty-two

"Good morning, Ansley, Savannah. Thank you for joining Aaron and I," said Kristian. "We have, shall we say, an interesting challenge confronting us. First, for Savannah's benefit, I will explain an effect of the transition to synthetic bodies that all who have transitioned have experienced. Savannah, all four of us have had a supernatural encounter that has led to several instances of literally saving humanity from extreme suffering." Kristian explained the encounters with the Guardian, including that involving the U.S. Civil War, World War II, The Cuban Missile Crisis, and the most recent—the Chinese virus threat of 2028.

Savannah sat silent, wide-eyed for at least a full minute, as Kristian concluded his description of their supernatural experiences and The Guardian. She then looked directly at Aaron and said, "You have experienced what Kristian has described?"

Aaron nodded and simply said, "Yes. Now listen carefully to what I am about to tell you. One encounter that Kristian did not describe was our travel forward in time to the year 2052." He described the threat that Find Corporation, along with two telecommunications giants, which was the ability to alter a person's reality and control their actions using a smartphone as a delivery vehicle of commands and images directly into the human brain. Aaron described the encounter, including how the cyborg spirits derailed the demonstration for the Secretary of Defense.

Kristian then raised the possibility of sabotaging the Find Corporation project to develop the technology necessary to facilitate what Aaron had just described. He concluded, "Does anyone have questions regarding what we've told you so far?"

After a few moments of silence, Savannah said with an emotional tone, "Please, give me a moment to comprehend what I've heard this morning. I mean, have I just crossed into The Twilight Zone?" referring to the 1960s television show of the same name. "Here I have three of the people that I respect most telling me about spirits, angels, time travel,… and mind control?"

Then Ansley spoke up, "Savannah, I reacted much in the same way the first time Kristian told me about his adventures with The Guardian. I nearly broke down thinking that my beloved husband, who had been through so much, was having a mental collapse. What he told me went against all of my scientific training and experience. But now I believe him. Given a little time, I think you will too. Please listen to the rest of this story."

After a few more silent moments, Savannah overcame her emotion, wiped a tear from her cheek and said, looking directly at Aaron, "OK, I am still in shock, but please continue. I need to know why this is being revealed to me now and not sooner."

Kristian continued, explaining his and Aaron's involvement in the early stages of the Kind Corporation project, including the meetings they had attended, the attendees, and the direction agreed to at the most recent meeting. He described the need to develop the wireless computer-brain interface that could target specific regions of the brain and plant images and commands that the subject would then execute. Kristian also said that he knew the U.S. military was involved in the development of this technology and it involved DARPA. The project, at least at this stage, appeared targeted for military use only. But, from their trip forward to 2052, plans were already set to use the technology to dominate the masses globally and completely control humanity. Kristian concluded with his volunteering of Savannah to take part, if not lead, in the technology's development and the development of a backdoor means of disabling the technology.

"Savannah, would you be willing to help us? This will require you to share the knowledge and information you have gained from your work with the human brain."

"Yes… I guess so. From the project that resulted in controlling a synthetic body using a human mind, we now have a highly detailed map of the functions of the brain and the locations, down to the cranial nerves, where all these functions reside. If, for example, we wanted to alter a subject's perception of the weather or introduce an odor, we know exactly where to target the commands. There are many nerves in the brain, known as cranial nerves, that handle various body functions and movements. Each nerve plays an individual role, but many of the nerves work together to perform more complicated bodily functions. Some nerves in the brain are the facial nerves, the trigeminal nerve, and the olfactory nerve. Some functions of the cranial nerves include chewing, eye movement, and facial sensations."

"Excellent," said Kristian. "It sounds like we already may know where to target the delivery of commands and images, as well as other sensory effects, provided a highly sophisticated delivery system can be developed around a smartphone interface. Do we know how the technology could be disabled on a massive scale, effectively preventing its use without damaging the subject's brain?"

"A rather primitive form of transmitting signals to the brain to effect a specified outcome has been done previously. Transmitting signals from the brain to prosthetics, for example, has been gaining sophistication over the past thirty years," said Savannah. "Just thinking about blocking this ability leads me to one possibility, introducing a virus, a computer virus, that would destroy the programs that issue and transmit the commands. Developing a virus would not be difficult. Introducing it into a highly secured program would be very difficult, but not impossible. Also, no doubt these programs would have sophisticated backup and disaster recovery, which would need to be considered. Otherwise, the programs could be restored in a matter of hours, or at most, days. Perhaps the virus could be introduced but lay dormant until sufficient backups that include the virus code are completed. Then, when activated, the virus would also destroy the backups."

"I would like you to attend the quarterly project status meeting with Aaron," said Kristian. "In the meantime, please continue investigating the possibility of introducing a virus that would disable the ability of the program to issue commands. From our trip into the future, it appears we have plenty of time, but we must diligently continue our efforts. Aaron, I am counting on you to monitor the other project team members for any revelation of evil intentions for the use of this technology. We must continue to develop alternative strategies in order to cancel what could prove to be the demise of freedom."

Chapter Twenty-three

December 17, 2042.

Erik and Ksenia arrived in Bergen, Norway, via Reykjavik, Iceland at approximately twelve noon. By the time they claimed their baggage, cleared Norwegian immigration, and got the rental car, it was a little after 1:00 PM local time. As they plotted their course to the Anderson estate in Flåm using their navigation app, all roads were shown as clear, with no ice or snow buildup. The navigation app showed they would arrive at the Anderson home at 5:13 PM.

The last time Erik had made the trip from Bergen to Flåm, it had been in May. Flåm was a lovely small town that sits at the end of Aurlandsfjord, a branch of the vast Sognefjord. The scenery along the fjords was breathtaking. Everything was fresh, renewed from the typical harsh winter of the region. This time, he saw that winter had already made its debut. Most of the landscape was covered in snow and the deciduous trees in the forests were bare. The fjords were still mostly free of ice, but the water seemed darker, as if it was warning one to stay on the shore. Erik attributed the darker water to the difference in the light cast by the sun at this time of year. As he drove, when Ksenia and he weren't talking, he kept rehearsing in his mind how he would tell Ksenia about his… condition. That she might reject him for any reason concerned him greatly.

"You're quiet today. Are you tired from the trip?" Ksenia asked.

"N… No. I just have some… things on my mind. Work stuff."

"Well, it's time to let that go and relax for the holidays," she said, rubbing his right leg.

"I know. It will still be there when I get back," said Erik.

It was dark when they arrived at the Anderson home shortly after 5 PM. As they pulled up to the house, Ksenia's parents and Thor, Ksenia's brother, came out to greet them.

"So wonderful to see you both again!" exclaimed Ebba, Ksenia's mother, as she hugged both Ksenia and Erik.

Erik, surprised at Ebba's greeting, chuckled and said, "thrilled to be here." He then turned to Carl, Ksenia's father, extending his hand and said, "Good to see you, sir."

"Good to see you, Erik," said Carl.

Thor, standing next to his father, extended his hand toward Erik and said, "Welcome back, Erik. We should have more time to talk this visit as my hours running the farm are much less this time of year. In the meantime, let me help you with your baggage."

"I'd like that, Thor," said Erik.

They then went inside into the living room, where a fire was burning in the fireplace. Ebba had prepared appetizers, pickled herring and crackers, and placed them on the coffee table. Carl began pouring vodka into shot-sized glasses.

"Everyone, please take a glass and I will give a toast," said Carl. In a moment, he raised his class, as did the others. "To the safe arrival of our sea-wandering daughter and her spaceship captain. May we always be together. "

To Erik, the depressing cloud following the death of Arya, Ksenia's sister, aboard the USS Elon Musk that had hung over the family on his last visit in May had faded. Their mood seemed lighter. Ebba appeared happier, as did Carl and even Thor, who had initially blamed Erik for Arya's death. The adage time heals appears to be true, he thought.

"This salmon is delicious," said Erik after taking his first bite of the dish served at dinner. "How do you make it, Mrs. Anderson?"

"Thank you, Erik. This dish is called Gravlaks, which is basically salmon that has been cured in salt, sugar, and dill. It is very popular with Norwegians."

At the conclusion of the meal, Carl said, rising from his chair at the head of the table, "Erik, Thor, come with me to the parlor for an after dinner drink while Ebba and Ksenia clean up."

Erik caught Ksenia glaring at her father after that remark and smirked at her, knowing he would never get away with such a statement. "Yes, sir," he said, looking directly at Ksenia, smiling.

As the three men sat, Carl said to Erik, "So your Board of Inquiry hearing went well?"

"Yes, sir. It was short. Over in less than ten minutes, and I was restored to flight status immediately."

"What does your navy have you doing now?" asked Thor.

"I have been assigned to a land-based role working with the development of… spacecraft enhancements. I am based at the Pentagon for now but will move to Nevada next year and will probably remain there for up to three years."

"What enhancements are you working on? Will you be developing technologies we've seen on Star Trek like warp drive and transporter?" asked Carl.

"Much of what I'll be working on is classified, but the projects should develop our ability to travel much further into deep space."

"Sounds quite interesting," said Carl.

Ksenia then came into the parlor carrying a tray of pastries. "Mother has prepared some very tempting desserts for us. Please enjoy!"

After a couple hours of friendly discussion on the state of the Anderson farming operation, Ksenia's cruises, the expected weather for the coming winter months, and Ebba's recipes, they retired for the evening.

On the way upstairs to the bedrooms, Erik asked Ksenia, "Let's take an early morning walk through the forest."

"Sounds good. But be sure to bundle up. The morning temperatures this time of year are below zero, centigrade or mid-twenties Fahrenheit. You'll also need proper boots as there is already snow on the ground. What time do you want to go? Daylight doesn't appear before nine thirty this time of year."

"Let's go around 9 AM and see if we can catch the sunrise."

Erik and Ksenia did not sleep together out of respect for Ksenia's parents. Each went to their respective bedroom after a goodnight kiss. Erik sat on the bed and opened his portable charging device and plugged the USB cord into the socket located under a flap of skin at the back of his neck. Recently, Ansley had provided a USB-sized plug to replace the bulky cable that he used previously. He lay down on his back and his mind immediately began rehearsing his talk planned for the next morning with Ksenia regarding his condition. What would he do if she could not accept the fact that his body was synthetic? How would the Andersons react if they saw she was upset? These thoughts plagued him off and on as he attempted to rest his mind and made the night excruciatingly long.

He looked at the clock on the nightstand several times during the night. The last time he looked at the clock, it said 5:42. By then, he had had enough rest and got up. He dressed and carried his shoes and laptop with him as he descended to the first floor. As he approached the parlor, he saw shadows of the flames from the fireplace flickering on the opposite wall. As he entered the room, he saw Carl sitting in his favorite chair.

"Erik, please come in. You are up early. Did you not sleep well?"

"I slept well, thank you. I believe it is just the time change. My body thinks it is still in LA time, noon," he said, chuckling. "Do you rise this early normally?"

"Yes, I'm usually up by five o'clock most mornings. Seems the older I get, the earlier I wake."

After a few moments of small talk, Carl returned to his laptop reading the news and Erik opened his to check email.

Carl then said, "have you seen this?" handing the laptop to Erik. What Erik saw caught him by complete surprise that didn't go unnoticed by Carl. A video was paused with the headline "SEVERLY INJURED NAVY PILOT SEEN CLIMBING INTO COCKPIT OF NAVY JET." The video showed Scarlett climbing a ladder up to the cockpit of a T-38. The video continued showing the jet beginning to taxi. It also showed the back of a male, presumed also to be a pilot, climbing into the rear seat of the jet. The male pilot had his helmet on so his face could not be seen from the back or side. The narrator said, "Navy pilot, Lt. Scarlett Bross, had been severely injured in an accident aboard the USS Trump in the South China Sea just months before. Records show she lost most of her left leg and left arm, which had to be amputated to save her life. How is it possible that she now appears whole and completely healed enough to fly a jet aircraft? We'll be investigating this story and will provide regular updates as information is obtained."

Erik, contemplating his response to Carl, sat silent for several moments. "I was not aware of this video report. I heard about Lt. Bross' accident and multiple amputations were performed to save her. How she appears to be completely healed in such a relatively short time is a mystery. In fact, I took over her training at the Barnett Center for Neurological Restoration in November and I was the male pilot you see climbing into the rear seat. That flight was her first flight since her accident."

"So, you know this pilot?"

"Yes, she appeared completely healed when I met her in November. I thought at the time that the reports of her injuries were grossly exaggerated. Also, they are doing some amazing… procedures with artificial limbs at Barnett Center."

Just then, Ksenia appeared. Erik called her to his side and replayed the video. "I didn't know that Scarlett had been so severely injured. I really know little about her condition after her accident.

The man climbing into the backseat of that jet looks like you. Is that you, Erik?"

"Yes, that's me. You remember when Scarlett and I went to Nevada a few weeks ago?"

"Yes, said Ksenia, frowning. I remember."

"I expect I will hear from Captain Barnes regarding this," said Erik.

"Will you have to return to Washington?" asked Ksenia.

"I hope not."

Ksenia then went into the kitchen to fix coffee for everyone and help Ebba get breakfast ready. In the meantime, Thor joined Carl and Erik in the parlor.

Everyone sat at the dining room table as Ebba and Ksenia served breakfast. After dining on a selection of yogurt, eggs, and oatmeal, Erik said, "Thank you for breakfast, Mrs. Anderson. Ksenia, the weather looks clear. Shall we go on our walk?"

Chapter Twenty-four

Just as Ksenia and Erik were stepping outside for their morning walk, Erik's phone emitted a sonar ping tone showing the incoming call was on a secure line. The caller ID said, "U.S. Department of Defense." Erik stopped and said, "I have to take this call," and picked up his smartphone.

"This is Commander Richards, to whom am I speaking?"

"Erik, this is Captain Barnes. Sorry to bother you on leave. Have you seen the videos of Scarlett Bross and you taking off in a Navy T-38?"

"Yes, sir. Just a few minutes ago."

"The brass, all the way up to SecDef, are breathing down my neck over this. I am going to a meeting with them in ten minutes. What do I tell them about Scarlett's miraculous recovery?"

"What I've told the folks here is that Barnett Center has been doing some astounding restoration of lost limbs. When I met her at the Center in November and assumed her recovery training, she appeared completely healed. I'm sure my sister Savannah could back you up on that."

Captain Barnes was silent for a few moments when he said, "But the brass already knows Scarlett is a… has a synthetic body."

"Yes, I know. What I gave you was a response that could be embellished to release to the press."

"You know that response would throw Barnett Center and Savannah under the bus with the media? They would be all over them seeking information on Barnett's restorative programs."

"Captain, that's the best response I have now. Barnett has a public relations department in place to deal with the media. They can handle it."

"Weak, Commander! What were you two doing going flying, anyway? We were nowhere near ready to release Scarlett back to the public."

"Following your orders, sir. Going to the meeting at Groom Lake, Area 51."

"OK, stay tuned and keep a bag packed. You may need to return to Washington sooner than either of us wants."

Chapter Twenty-five

Ksenia and Erik began their walk through the forest surrounding the house. The snow on the ground was powdery and the air a cold twenty-four degrees Fahrenheit. They saw a red fox standing still, looking directly at them. As they stepped toward it, it ran off through the woods.

"Was that Captain Barnes? From your tone, it sounds like people are getting excited over Scarlett flying with you?" said Ksenia.

"Typical response anytime the media are involved and are questioning the higher-ups. Everyone is looking for a place to point their finger to deflect the wrath away from themselves."

As they came upon the shore of a lake, they stopped. Erik turned to face Ksenia and held her shoulders in his hands. "I have something very important to share with you. It is the main reason that I asked you to sign those non-disclosure commitments for the government."

"OK," she said.

"I never want to keep anything about me from you. And I believe you feel the same way. There is one thing, one very important thing about me you must know."

"O… K… please go on," said Ksenia, growing concern clear in her voice, her green eyes looking directly into Erik's.

"You know I was involved in a terrible accident aboard my spaceship. All the doctors said I would never walk again, that I would have very limited mobility of my hands and arms. I would spend the rest of my life in a wheelchair. What you don't know is how I could recover and resume a normal life."

"Yes, I thought it was the miracle cures at the Barnett Center that revived you like they revived Scarlett."

"Well, that's partially true. But those cures were much more than cures. I am now in a completely new, synthetic body. This body you see is not flesh and bones. It is synthetic materials molded together that my mind, uploaded from my broken body and downloaded to this body, occupies."

Ksenia's eyes widened as she said, "You're not joking, are you?"

"No, Ksenia. I am not. As you already know from the time we have spent together that this body is fully functional in every way. In fact, it exceeds human functionality. I have the strength of ten men and can run at speeds exceeding sixty miles per hour. But the most important part is that I have all the emotions of a normal human man."

After several moments of silence, Ksenia took a step backwards, tears welling up in her eyes. "You are telling me you are a… robot?"

"No, I am not telling you that. I am telling you I am a loving, caring human mind dwelling in a synthetic body. Look, what if I had artificial arms or legs? Would I still be human or something less because I only had part of a human body?"

She thought about that last statement for a few moments. "This explains some feats I've seen you perform since we've been going together. That time you nearly threw me up to the ceiling at my flat in Bergen. Or that day on the beach in Ocean City when you rescued that girl trapped in the undertow. Even that thick metal towel bar you broke in our hotel room."

"Yes, that was me getting used to my new body and learning how to control my strength."

"I didn't know you before your accident. But I believe you when you say that your mind, your human mind, is… controlling your body. You aren't an advanced android like… who was that character on Star Trek?"

"Mr. Data."

"Yes, Mr. Data. So, are you the only living person with a synthetic body?

"No. Kristian, Aaron, and Scarlett all are synthetics."

Ksenia stepped back from Erik, contemplating all that she had just heard. "That means that Ansley is happily married to a synthetic human. And isn't Savannah dating Aaron?"

"Exactly," said Erik. "Ansley especially knows there is no difference in Kristian's mind or how he cares for her. She married him when he was… not synthetic."

Ksenia then turned back to Erik and reached up to touch his face. "Your skin feels… human. Your eyes look human."

Erik took her hand and said, "I am human. I have a human mind, as I always have. Science has enabled the cure of my nearly dead body. It is simply an advancement of science that routinely replaces limbs and organs with synthetics. In my case, as well as the other three, my entire body was replaced."

Their conversation continued as they resumed their walk around the lake.

"Will you age like a normal human?" asked Ksenia.

"This body will not age. Ansley can give me some appearances of aging, like graying and thinning my hair or adding wrinkles to my skin."

"So, theoretically you can live forever?"

"Theoretically, that would seem to be the case. But what will not be known for some time is how my human mind will adapt to a life span of indefinite length. That won't be known for decades as we synthetics age."

"Then, as I age, you will not. When I am an old woman, wrinkled and slow with gray hair, you will still be the way you are now."

"Ansley can make me look old."

"What happens if you… your synthetic body is destroyed? You could be in an accident, a plane crash or something."

"My mind is not only stored in this body, but a backup copy is stored in multiple databases across the globe. For security reasons, multiple copies are stored in different locations. In the event this body is destroyed, my mind could be downloaded to a new body. That briefcase you see me carrying whenever we travel is a backup and charging device. The batteries powering my body, located where kidneys would normally be found, are good for about seventy-two hours. So I must regularly charge them."

"But you eat and drink like a human."

"I eat and drink for social reasons and simple pleasures. My body disposes of anything I consume. I do not experience hunger and alcohol has no effect on me."

"I am getting cold. Let's head back to the house and grab a cup of hot chocolate," said Ksenia.

After a few moments of silence, "Has anything I have told you changed the way you feel about… us?" said Erik.

"No. In fact, I am glad you had the… courage to tell me. You didn't know how I would react, yet you told me anyway."

"I admit, I have had concerns about telling you for some time. I certainly didn't want to lose you. But I felt strongly that if we were to continue to develop our relationship, that you must know."

Just then, a snowball hit Ksenia on the back of her shoulder. They both turned to see Thor laughing at them. Erik picked up snow and formed a snowball and hurled it at Thor. Thor ducked, still laughing when Ksenia's snowball hit him in the face as he bent down. Fortunately, the powdery snow inflicted no injury.

"No fair, two against one!" yelled Thor.

They then turned, laughing, to return to the house together.

Chapter Twenty-six

Monday, December 22, 2042. 11:00 AM. The Pentagon.

The Pentagon press briefing began with comments from Andrew Fitzpatrick, Press Secretary. A summary of military activities across the globe ensued, with its usual emphasis on Chinese exercises in the South China Sea. The United States was still monitoring the Chinese after the takeover of Taiwan in 2024, enabled by the weak and ineffective Biden administration which blocked retaliatory U.S. military intervention and capitulated to Chinese President Xi. The U.S. Navy still maintained a presence in the region, re-established after Donald Trump's reelection in 2024, currently with the aircraft carrier USS Donald Trump. Threats were regularly exchanged between China and the United States pertaining to the U.S. involvement in allegedly sponsoring resistance to the Communist Chinese on the island state.

The Press Secretary then opened the floor to questions. Several questions referenced military activities in Asia and in Afghanistan, where militant extremists had been challenging the Taliban's rule established in 2021. References to involvement by the CIA in supporting the resistance were deflected. The Press Secretary simply referred the questioners to the CIA.

Then a question came from a correspondent for Fox News: "Mr. Secretary, regarding the video of just a few days ago showing Lt. Scarlett Bross and Commander Erik Richards taking off in a Navy jet, how does the Pentagon explain their miraculous recoveries?"

"I don't believe I would characterize their recoveries as miraculous," replied Fitzpatrick. "They both had serious injuries that were recoverable."

"Commander Richards' injuries aboard the USS Musk were widely publicized as resulting in serious permanent disability, as were Lt. Bross'."

"I am not familiar with the details of their respective cases. I can say that they were both treated at the Barnett Center for Neurological Restoration in California." The Secretary then pointed to another reporter who had raised her hand, cutting off the Fox News correspondent from further questions.

Later, the same day, Barnett Center public relations began receiving media inquiries regarding Erik's and Scarlett's treatments and recovery. A press release was issued quoting Barnett Industries CEO Noel Donovan. "The Barnett Center for Neurological Restoration has been the world leader in neurological restoration and artificial prostheses for decades. The cure for Alzheimer's disease was developed by Dr. Savannah Richards and her team. Since then, Dr. Richards has pioneered the continued development of artificial limbs for the human body. The surgical techniques and devices used specifically for Commander Erik Richards and Lt. Scarlett Bross are classified and will not be discussed further."

Questions from news organizations continued to flood Barnett Public Relations but went unanswered. In the meantime, smartphone video footage of Erik's rescue of the teenage girl in the surf at Ocean City, Maryland was released by CNN. Accompanying the footage was a caption stating Erik's speed running into the surf was clocked at thirty-four miles per hour. The video also captured Erik's response to a question by a lifeguard regarding his performance: "I'm in the Navy."

Later in the day, Erik received a classified message from Naval Space Command: "Change of Orders for Commander Erik Richards. Effective 05 January 2043, Report to Nellis AFB, Nevada, to continue current assignments."

Erik messaged Captain Barnes to confirm the new orders. Barnes replied, "The Pentagon brass felt it was important to get you as far away from the media spotlight as possible. Scarlett received the same orders. You both will be stationed at Nellis until the new facilities at Groom Lake can be completed. SecDef wanted you stationed at Space Dock, but we talked him down from that, given the need to have you continue your current project."

Erik then went to update Ksenia, who was in the kitchen helping Ebba with lunch. "Ksenia, my orders were changed. I now must report to Nellis Air Force Base on January fifth. I will not be returning to the Pentagon. I will be stationed at Nellis until our new facilities at Groom Lake are completed."

"Was this a result of the events in the news? What will that mean for my leave scheduled to begin in April?" asked Ksenia.

"Yes. The Pentagon brass were spooked by the likelihood of paparazzi descending on the Pentagon and wanted me as far away from them as possible. I guess I'm lucky they didn't send me out to sea or up to Space Dock. I'm sure we'll be able to work something out when you go on leave."

Chapter Twenty-seven

Christmas Eve, 2042.

Erik rose early. He had been dwelling most of the night on how to propose to Ksenia today. But first, he must get with Carl, Ksenia's father, to ask for his blessing for the proposal. He quietly descended the stairs at around 5:30 and saw that Carl was up and seated in his usual spot in the parlor.

"Good morning, Mr. Anderson. I hope this Christmas Eve finds you well," said Erik.

"Good morning, Erik. Please join me here by the fire."

"Sir, I have something I need to ask of you."

"Oh? Please, what can I do for you, Erik?"

"I would like to ask for your blessing to ask Ksenia for her hand in marriage. We have been together for seven months and our love for each other continues to grow."

"When do you intend to propose to her?"

"Today. With your blessing, of course."

"Do you have any concerns committing to each other, given you are separated for months at a time?"

"So far, we have dealt with the times we are separated without problems," said Erik.

"Erik, you have mine and Ebba's blessing. We couldn't ask for a better man for our daughter."

"Thank you, sir," Erik said, smiling.

It was a cold, crisp, clear morning as Ksenia and Erik stepped outside for their morning walk through the woods. The snowfall over the past two-days lay down a pure white thirteen-inch blanket over the land that was beautiful but added a challenge to walking. The two proceeded into the woods towards the lakeshore where they first kissed. As they came up to the shore, Ksenia a bit out of breath because of the deep snow, Erik turned to face her, grabbing her gloved hands, and kneeled. He withdrew a small black velvet box from his coat pocket, opened it, and held it up to Ksenia.

"Ksenia, I think you know I love you deeply. I truly cannot imagine my life without you. Will you marry me?"

Ksenia momentarily looked up at the sky, tears forming, then looked down into Erik's azure blue eyes. "Y... Yes!" she exclaimed.

Erik then stood and removed the mitten on Ksenia's left hand, and placed the 3.01 carat GIA certified, G-SI2, round diamond, flanked by round brilliant diamonds on each side on her ring finger. The two embraced and kissed for what seemed like several minutes.

"This ring is beautiful, Erik! It must have set you back thousands of dollars." Erik paid over $76,000 for the ring, which, according to the saleswoman, was a terrific price.

"When I first saw the ring, it jumped right out at me, saying it was made especially for you. I couldn't resist."

They continued their walk around the lake, occasionally stopping to rest after trudging through the deep snow when Ksenia said, "you said you cannot imagine your life without me in it. Will you feel the same when I am old and wrinkled? Or when I pass away? Or is there a way I could become... immortal like you?"

"Hopefully, it will be many years before we will face our old age. Perhaps by then, life extension with good health will be available," said Erik.

Back at the manor house, Carl went into the Kitchen where Ebba was preparing their Christmas feast. "Ebba, I have some news to share with you."

"Oh?" Ebba replied.

"Erik is proposing to Ksenia today. He came to me this morning to ask for my blessing."

"Oh, my!" exclaimed Ebba, turning to face Carl. "Our baby girl is getting married…," as tears welled up in her eyes. "Have you told Thor?"

"No, I will let them tell Thor."

"I hope he takes it well," said Ebba.

"I think he will. He's been quite friendly with Erik since Erik and Ksenia arrived."

When Ksenia and Erik arrived back at the manor house, Ksenia, glowing both from the cold and the events of the morning, went straight into the kitchen, where Ebba was working on their Christmas celebration. She removed the mitten from her left hand and held it out to Ebba. Ebba, pretending she knew nothing, looked at the hand and gasped.

"Is… Is this what it appears to be, Ksenia?"

"Yes, mother," she replied, throwing her arms around Ebba. "Erik and I are to be married!"

"That is quite a ring!" exclaimed Ebba. "He must have paid thousands."

"He said that he couldn't limit his love," said Ksenia.

"What a beautiful response. Ksenia, your father and I believe you have found the best man you could. Hang on to him. Do not let him get away," said Ebba, smiling and looking directly into her daughter's eyes. "Do you know when you will be wed?"

"Not yet, Momma. But I hope it will be soon."

"Will you tell Thor?"

"We will make an announcement at Christmas dinner this evening. Please don't tell him before."

"Your father insisted that you and Erik tell Thor and forbade me to say anything."

"So, Father knew Erik was going to propose?"

"Yes, he told me that Erik came to him this morning to ask for his blessing to propose to you."

"But he didn't know I would accept."

"Dear, your father and I both could see the love you have for Erik. He knew you would accept."

Later that afternoon, Erik and Ksenia video-called the Barnett mansion where Erik's and Savannah's parents were spending Christmas.

"Dad, Mom, Savannah, I… We have an announcement to make. Ksenia and I are engaged to be married!"

"That's wonderful," said Erik's mother.

"Congratulations!" said his father.

"Wow! Ksenia, we'll have to get together so I can share all of Erik's secrets with you," said Savannah, smiling.

"Thanks for the warning, sis!" said Erik. "I will prepare Ksenia before you two meet and Savannah disparages me."

Erik then motioned to Carl and Ebba, who were off camera. "Here are Ksenia's parents," as he turned the camera towards them.

"Happy Christmas," said Carl.

"It is happy, indeed," said Ebba. "We are thrilled with Erik."

"He is thrilled with you as well," said Erik's mother.

After several minutes of chatting back and forth, the call ended with a round of Christmas wishes.

Christmas Eve ended at the Anderson home with a traditional Christmas dinner of pinnekjøtt–dried mutton ribs, swede mash (rotmos), which comprises carrots and potatoes, and lingonberry jam.

Chapter Twenty-eight

December 28, 2042, 3:12 AM
Barnett Mansion, Bel-Air, California

Kristian was in a deeply relaxed state when he saw a mist form in his mind. Ansley was fast asleep at his side. As he gained consciousness, he saw the shape of The Guardian form as the mist receded.

"Guardian, you have come in need of my abilities to influence critical decisions affecting humanity?"

"Yes, Kristian. We have a timeline that has gone astray in the recent past. If not corrected, the changes will dramatically affect the future from that point forward, including the present."

"Recent past?" said Kristian, as he realized his spirit had exited the synthetic body resting next to Ansley.

"Yes, grab hold of my arm and I will provide the details. We will raise Erik as well and bring him with us."

In an instant, Kristian and Erik find themselves in a Chinese munitions factory. The Guardian points out rows of missiles hanging in racks from the ceiling.

"Gentlemen, the date is January 6, 2024. What you see above you are one hundred hypersonic missiles capable of delivering nuclear bombs anywhere on the planet. These missiles travel in low-Earth orbit at speeds up to twenty-one thousand miles per hour. They can evade virtually every detection system available. The Chinese Communist Party is planning to threaten the United States and the European Union with annihilation if the U.S. does not capitulate to their demands. Party Chairman and President Xi Jinping have generated a letter detailing the demands of the CCP to President Joe Biden."

The Guardian continued, "There are two potential outcomes from this blatant act of aggression against the West. First, if the U.S. capitulates to the Chinese demands, China will militarily take control of the entire Far East. Taiwan will fall immediately. Japan, Australia, and New Zealand will fall soon after. With the U.S. capitulating, the Canada and the European Union stand down. Great Britain is furious with the U.S. as its Commonwealth nations in the Pacific are now certain to fall. Singapore and Thailand are also targeted by China and expected to surrender. India and Pakistan will ultimately fall to Chinese rule. Even Russian President Vladimir Putin believes Russia is threatened by Chinese aggression. Within two years of U.S. capitulation, China controls the entire Pacific region and is, indeed, threatening Eastern Russia."

"There can be only one future as China continues to expand its domain. China will continue to grow in power until it is unstoppable. They will use their nuclear and missile superiority to force the surrender of all Middle Eastern and European nations. China will control the supply of oil to Europe, and to North and South America. Thanks to President Biden's deliberate policies leading to failure to maintain independence and control of the supply of oil established under President Donald Trump, the U.S. economy experiences an unprecedented depression as all economic activity comes to a halt. Millions of Americans, mostly in large urban and suburban areas, are literally dying of starvation and disease. In the end, China quickly establishes control over the entire planet. In Europe, India, and the Middle East, people of races other than Asian are gathered and forced into concentration camps where living conditions are abysmal. In India and the Middle East, the camps exist for the termination of several billion people so that there is room for the growing Asian horde. In the end, what is left of humanity that is not of the Asian race is thrown into perpetual medieval slavery and worse."

"Guardian, did the United States or Russia perhaps have any similar weapon with which to counter the Chinese hypersonic missile?" asked Kristian.

"The short answer is no," replied Erik. "During the Trump presidency, development of hypersonic missile capability that compared favorably to the Chinese technology was nearly completed. But the Biden administration that followed decimated funding for military research and development. When Donald Trump was elected for a second term in 2024, followed by Ron DeSantis in 2028, and the U.S. Congress was fully controlled by the Republican Party of the time, significant funding went for the continued development of hypersonic missile capability. By 2032, we had matched the nuclear capability of the Chinese. In addition, systems that could detect and destroy hypersonic missiles were developed and deployed, effectively eliminating any threat by the Chinese or any other nation that developed the technology."

"Guardian, you mentioned two scenarios with different outcomes," said Kristian.

"Yes, and it is the second scenario where you and Erik will play a pivotal role. Take my arm again, both of you."

The three spirits instantaneously found themselves in The Cabinet Room of the White House. Present were President Joe Biden, Vice President Kamala Harris, Secretary of State Anthony Blinken, Secretary of Defense Lloyd Austin, Director of the CIA William Burns, Director of Homeland Security Alejandro Mayorkas, and the Joint Chiefs of Staff. Also notably present were former President Barack Obama and White House Director of Domestic Policy Council Susan Rice.

"Mr. President," began Chairman of the Joint Chiefs General Mark Milley. "We, the Joint Chiefs, agree that we must refuse the

Chinese ultimatum. Frankly, sir, we believe the Chinese are bluffing. Yes, they have the nuclear missiles, but they know using them on the United States would be suicide. We should instead go to Defcon 2."

"Remind me again what Defcon 2 specifies," mumbles Biden.

"Defcon 2 is declared when intelligence findings indicate a risk for an impending attack, such as the case in the Cuban missile crisis in 1962," said General Milley.

"Director Burns, do your intelligence sources show we are in a situation demanding Defcon 2?" asked Vice President Harris.

"Yes, Madame Vice President," replied Burns.

"Mr. President," began Secretary Blinken. "The United States has no means to stop the Chinese. The only sign we have of a launch of their hypersonic missiles is real-time satellite photos of their many launch sites throughout China. And then we have no way of knowing where these missiles are pointed. If we capitulate to their demands, we can preserve the peace indefinitely."

Biden, wide-eyed, turned to look directly at former President Obama. "Barack, what do you recommend? What would you do?"

"Joe, until now, we have had a good relationship with China and President Xi. Giving up our presence in the Pacific is a relatively small price to pay to achieve a lasting peace with them," said Barack Obama.

"President Obama, giving up our presence in the Pacific will cause the immediate fall of Taiwan. Japan and Australia will be threatened. Hell, even Hawaii could be taken," said Director Burns, his disdain for Obama's reply to Biden's question clear.

"Mr. President, you have our staff recommendation to capitulate to the Chinese. Our review of the situation shows China will want to maintain world trade. If they exercise excess aggression, trade with both the E.U. and the U.S. will be threatened. Canada has already stated their support for capitulation," said Susan Rice.

"Capitulation will cause the continued erosion of U.S. sovereignty," said Defense Secretary Austin. "A significant number of Americans will consider this treason. Millions will believe that capitulation will make the botched Afghanistan withdrawal pale in comparison."

"So, we deliberately goad the Chinese into annihilating us by rejecting their proposal?" said Secretary Blinken, his voiced raised.

The room grew silent as all saw Biden put his head in his hands for what seemed much longer than it was. "Why are the Chinese taking this position now, at the end of my presidency?" he mumbled.

"Sir, the Chinese fear that Donald Trump will regain the White House in November. They know he would never capitulate to their demands," said Secretary Mayorkas.

"Gentlemen," said Biden as he raised his head to face them, ignoring the women in the room. "Let's keep this discussion civil. Susan, what do the polls say regarding how the voters feel about this issue?"

"Uh, sir, the public knows nothing of the Chinese demands," replied Rice.

"Oh… right," said Biden, the look on his face showing he was fading from stress and exhaustion, not to mention his declining cognitive state.

"I want a speech to the American people written. Actually, I want two speeches. One will state we are capitulating to the Chinese to maintain world peace. The other will indicate that we are not and that we are preparing our military defenses to prepare for possible Chinese aggression. Susan, get with our Press Secretary and schedule a prime-time TV delivery for 7:00 PM tomorrow evening from the Oval Office. This meeting is adjourned."

Biden then rose from his chair at the center of the table and walked slowly, slightly bent over, to the door as the room remained silent. As Biden exited the room, someone whispered, "God help us. We don't know what he will do tomorrow night."

"We must plan to ensure that Biden delivers the second speech," said The Guardian to Kristian and Erik.

"But won't taking a hard stance against the Chinese result in a nuclear holocaust?" asked Kristian.

"Perhaps, but we know capitulation will destroy humanity," replied The Guardian.

Chapter Twenty-nine

January 26, 2024, The Oval Office, 5:13 PM

Kristian, Erik, and The Guardian observe the activity setting up the Oval Office for President Biden's address to the nation. Three TV cameras face the President's desk. The middle camera contains the teleprompter screen from which Biden will read his speech. For speeches made from the Oval Office, all three cameras typically have teleprompters. But Biden often gets confused when facing over one teleprompter, repeating lines or skipping lines altogether. Two boom mikes hang out of sight of the cameras. Across from the desk, a technician is preparing to load Biden's speech into the teleprompter system. The speech Biden has ordered to be loaded details the plans for capitulation to the Chinese.

"Erik, you will need to enter the mind of the technician who is loading the speech into the teleprompter. You will direct him to load the second speech that calls for refusing to agree to the Chinese demands. Kristian, when President Biden delivers the speech, you will take control of Biden's mind and read the speech from the teleprompter. Since you will use Biden's voice, your control of Biden's mind will go unnoticed. If Biden appears to react to you taking control of his mind, it will be viewed as just one more stumble by Biden. When you are finished, the cameras will be shut off and you can exit Biden's mind."

"Guardian, Biden appears to suffer from dementia and impaired cognitive abilities. Will taking control of his mind cause a more severe reaction than we have seen in healthy minds?"

"It is possible that a more severe reaction could occur. But should Biden pass out or worse, the speech will be stopped, anyway. It is a risk that must be taken."

Erik moves closer to the technician preparing the teleprompter that will be attached to the middle TV camera. He notices the technician has a small black box about the size of a wristwatch box. The box is open on the desk where he is working and contains two USB drives, one colored red and one green. Picking up his secure phone, he calls an unknown party. He asks which USB to load into the teleprompter. As he picks up the green USB. Erik enters the technician's mind and takes control. The technician looks blankly at the green USB in his hand. He then puts it back in the black box and picks up the red USB. He inserts the red USB into the teleprompter control unit and uploads the speech. Erik sees a brief portion of the text on the teleprompter and verifies it is the correct speech. He exits the technician's mind as the technician takes the control unit and mounts it on the TV camera directly facing Biden. The technician then takes his laptop and the wristwatch box and leaves the Oval Office.

7:10 PM.

Joe Biden takes his seat at the presidential desk. Looking at the camera directly facing him, he sees the red light go to green. "Good evening. It is with grave concern I speak with my fellow Americans." At that moment, Kristian takes control of Biden's mind. Biden's eyes noticeably close for a couple of seconds. Whispers of "what's he doing?" are heard among the television staff present.

Kristian then delivers the speech through Biden. "We have received a verified communique from Beijing. The United States is being ordered out of the Far East and Pacific Region by China. President Xi Jinping has stated that China will aggressively attack the United States and her allies using their nuclear capable hypersonic missiles if we do not capitulate to their demands. In response, I have ordered our military to escalate to Defcon 2. Defcon 2 is declared when intelligence findings show a risk for an impending attack, such as the case during the Cuban missile crisis in 1962. Defcon 2 also calls for preparing our nuclear arsenal, both land and sea based, for launch."

Those watching the broadcast from The White House Situation Room, including the Vice President, Secretary of State, the Joint Chiefs, and former president Obama, are stunned. Just an hour prior, Biden had told them he was giving the speech to capitulate.

"Madame Vice President," said Secretary Blinken, "what has happened here? He's up there threatening our very existence with annihilation on global television! What can we do to stop this?"

"I... I'm afraid there is nothing we can do," replied Kamala Harris.

Pointing at the Joint Chiefs who were sitting together across the table from Harris, Obama, and Blinken, Blinken screamed, "You pulled this off? You got to Biden and convinced him to do this behind our backs!"

Kristian, again through Biden, continued, "We do not take this stance easily. Indeed, our very existence is threatened. But it would be markedly worse to capitulate to the egregious aggression of the Chinese Communists. We do not know how the Chinese Communists will react to our position. We pray they will come to their senses and realize that a nuclear attack will also result in their demise. In the meantime, we all must pray that God will continue to bless this nation. Thank you, and good night."

As Kristian left the mind of Joe Biden, Biden leaned over and put his face down in his hands for several moments. The TV cameras continued to record this reaction. When he raised his head, he stood up slowly and shuffled as he walked towards the exit of the Oval Office. The TV staff stood silent, in shock, as they viewed Biden's unsteady exit aided by the two Secret Service agents.

Outside the Oval Office, those that had been present in the Situation Room ambushed Biden. "What the hell do you think you were doing giving that speech, Joe?" said Obama with clear anger.

"Mr. President, do you realize that this could mean our annihilation?" asked Kamala Harris?

"Did the Joint Chiefs get to you, Mr. President, and get you to change your mind?" demanded Secretary Blinken.

"I… I don't know what happened. I thought I gave the order to load the speech to capitulate. I… frankly, don't have any idea what I just said on television. I… I need to lie down," stuttered Biden as he fell, only to be caught by the Secret Service agent standing at his side. The agent then led him towards the Presidential Bedroom on the second floor of the White House.

"We need to invoke the 25th Amendment immediately!" said Secretary Blinken. "It is the only action available that will save the country, indeed, the world! We can have a vote of the Cabinet within twenty-four hours. Kamala will be acting president and can reverse this planet-ending decision!"

Over the next several hours, communiques were received from multiple ally nations. Literally all expressed their admiration for Biden, expressing strength in his resistance to Chinese aggression. Great Britain, Australia, Japan, and the European Union countries all pledged to support the United States against China. International support for Biden effectively derailed any action towards invoking the Twenty-Fifth Amendment.

Chapter Thirty

In the Chinese Communist Party (CCP) offices in Beijing, it was 8:30 AM, the day after President Joe Biden rejected the Chinese demands for surrendering the Pacific. Beijing is thirteen hours ahead of U.S. East Coast time. Xi Jinping, CCP and State Military Commissions Chairman, and President is meeting with Fan Changlong, Vice Chairman of the CCP and State Military Commissions and Army General, and Xu Qiliang, Vice Chairman of the CCP and State Military Commissions and Air Force General. Unknown to these gentlemen was the presence of three spirits: The Guardian, Kristian, and Erik.

"Now that Biden has uncharacteristically refused to accept our terms, what shall be our strategy?" asked President Xi of his two top generals. "The rest of the western world has sided with Biden's decision and vowed to support the United States. This was totally unexpected given the intelligence we received regarding Biden."

The two generals looked at each other for a few moments, then General Changlong replied. "If we follow through with our threat of nuclear intervention to achieve our goals, we will risk annihilation of the entire planet. Even if they do not know where our missiles will strike, they will know they are launched with their orbital satellites.

And our missiles will do nothing to take out their nuclear missile equipped ships and submarines. The United States is at Defcon 2, which means they could launch their nukes before ours could strike."

"But if we do not follow through on our demands, we will look weak," said General Qiliang. "We could strike Hawaii, Alaska, and the United States West Coast cities in less than ten minutes from launching our missiles. A limited attack may encourage them to meet our demands."

"What is the percentage of their suborbital missiles that we could block using our defense shield should they launch in retaliation?" asked Xi Jinping.

"Approximately 80%, based on our testing," replied Qiliang.

"Whether we launch a limited strike or a full strike, the response would likely be their entire nuclear arsenal," said General Changlong.

"Perhaps we should launch a single unarmed missile, and have it circle the Earth as we did in 2021. This would express our displeasure in their rejection and a reminder of the power behind our demands. They will only see one launch from their satellite, which will make them hesitate to unleash their nuclear inventory on us," said General Changlong.

"I do not believe such saber-rattling will have much effect now that their allies have indicated they will stand behind them. At this point, I would prefer to embarrass them," said Xi. "What if we said that the communique they claim came from the CCP was actually a forgery, likely committed by their own intelligence agencies attempting to ignite a war with China? The Chinese Communist Party supports world peace and the reaction of the United States to the false communique resulted from weak intelligence by the Biden administration."

"This could be the best course of action," said General Changlong. "It would allow the current heightened state of arms to cool to a point where we could launch an attack without warning."

"It would also result in the allies of the United States to look once more with reduced trust in the Biden administration," said General Qiliang.

"So, we weaken the United States on the world stage once again without firing a shot," said Xi, smiling. "Are we in agreement?"

Both generals indicated they were.

"Guardian, has the crisis passed?" asked Kristian.

"For now, but there will always be another."

The reaction of the United States' allies worldwide was unified condemnation of the weak and ineffective actions of the Biden administration. Calls, both within and outside of the U.S., for Biden's resignation resonated through the halls of government in Washington, D.C. Statements by the Biden Administration calling the Chinese Communist Party response to Biden's accusations a lie further eroded confidence in the United States by its allies. Articles of Impeachment were drawn, voted and approved by the Republican majority in the House of Representatives. A trial ensued in the Senate that resulted in Biden's acquittal of high crimes and misdemeanors by a vote of sixty-two for and thirty-eight against, failing to achieve the required sixty-six votes to convict and remove Biden from office. Ten Democrats voted with all fifty-two Republicans to convict.

Biden canceled his campaign, already in progress, to run for a second term and finished the rest of his disastrous presidential term in disgrace.

Chapter Thirty-one

May 22, 2043, Bergen, Norway

Erik and Ksenia were wed aboard the Viking Cruise Lines Ship, Viking Sky. Wedding guests included Ksenia's parents, Carl and Ebba, and brother Thor. Erik's parents, Kristen and Edward, and sister Savannah were aboard, as were Kristian and Ansley Barnett, with their daughter, Kristen Elaine. Viking granted an exception to its no person under the age of eighteen policy at Kristian's request. Aaron Adams was also present. Captain Jeffrey Barnes, Erik's commanding officer, who was invited but could not attend, sent his best wishes to the couple, along with a lovely gift. Several of Ksenia's crewmates, with whom she had sailed on multiple cruises, were in attendance.

Ksenia's wedding dress was a glamorous mermaid silhouette, which amplified her curves for a sultry result. An elongated bodice hugged her body, and the skirt flared out at mid-thigh, creating an hourglass effect.

The ship departed Bergen for its first port-of-call in Flam, Norway, near Ksenia's home. Once the ship's captain assumed command from the harbor pilot, the wedding party gathered in the ship's Star Theater on Deck 2. Leaving his first officer in command of the bridge, the captain joined the wedding shortly following the party.

The captain, wearing a formal Viking Cruise Line captain's uniform, took his place on the theater stage facing the guests. Erik, dressed in formal U.S. Navy uniform, climbed the temporary stairs placed for the wedding in the middle of the stage, and took his place next to the ship's captain. Thor, Erik's best man, then joined the two already on the stage. Next to enter the theater was Ksenia's maiden of honor, Savannah, followed by Kristen Elaine as the flower girl. As a traditional Norwegian wedding march, performed by the Berntsons, played over the theater speakers, all heads turned towards the theater entrance where Ksenia and her father, Carl, began walking down the left aisle towards the stage. Seeing Ksenia for the first time in her wedding dress, Erik was momentarily breathless. Ksenia and Carl mounted the theater stage and stood in front of the captain.

"Who gives this woman in matrimony?" asked the captain.

"Her mother and I do," said Carl. Ksenia then took her place next to Erik as Carl then descended the steps and took his seat next to Ebba in the first row.

Erik and Ksenia recited their vows and were declared husband and wife by the captain. A reception followed in The Chef's Table, one of the ship's specialty restaurants. Tables were set in a buffet and offered delicacies from around the world, courtesy of Viking's renown head chef. An open bar offered top shelf liquor and a selection of fine wines to the guests. As best man, Thor gave a speech which contained a humorous recount of when Erik and Thor first met a year ago. Then Carl, Ksenia's father, gave a speech welcoming Erik and his family into the Anderson family. Finally, Edward spoke about how thrilled they were that Erik had brought Ksenia into the Richards family. When it came time for Erik and Ksenia to leave the reception, Ksenia tossed her bridal bouquet directly to Savannah.

As a wedding gift, Kristian and Ansley paid for Erik and Ksenia's accommodations in the ship's Owner's Suite which featured a King-size Viking Explorer bed with luxury linens, large flat-screen LCD

TV, mini-bar with complimentary alcoholic beverages, soft drinks, water & snacks, replenished daily, in-suite binoculars, coffee maker & cashmere blanket, luxury robes, slippers & toiletries, direct dial satellite phone & cell service, security safe, hair dryer, 110/220 volt outlets, complimentary Wi-Fi, and a bottle of champagne. The oversized suite was also used for small gatherings of the wedding party periodically throughout the cruise.

The entire wedding party continued the cruise, which saw several ports in Norway, the Faroe Islands, and Iceland, where the party disembarked in Reykjavik.

Chapter Thirty-two

Several days into the cruise, Erik and Ksenia were sitting outside on the Aquavit Terrace near the infinity pool when Ksenia said, "I am thinking about my future. Do I continue my career with Viking and sacrifice large portions of my time with you? Or should I give up that career and life, and come to be with you?"

"I thought we had agreed that you would continue your career until the time comes for children," said Erik with a questioning look on his face.

"We had. But I don't want to be separated for months at a time, several times per year. Long-distance relationships don't have an outstanding track record."

"If you joined me full time, what would you do while I was working? The project I'm working on requires extended hours to meet firm deadlines."

"What exactly is the project you're working on? Is there an opportunity for me to work with you?"

"Wow! I don't know." Erik took her hand and said, "I can disclose that to you now that we're married and you have your top-secret clearance," said Erik. "We are designing and building Earth's first starship."

"You… you are building what?" said Ksenia, her eyebrows raised and smiling. "Are you joking with me, Erik?"

"No joke. We are using information gathered over the past seventy years from unidentified aerial phenomena, UAPs, that were captured to design and build the first deep space exploratory vehicle. I am the Navy's project manager and have a staff of scientists and engineers. Scarlett is in astronaut training now, preparing for duty on the project and on the ship when it is launched. I hope to be the ship's captain when it is ready for launch."

Following a few moments of silence, Ksenia, her Norwegian accent growing thicker indicating she was becoming emotional, then asked, "So what happens to me when you fly off to the stars? How long would you be gone? Scarlett would be a crew member…?"

"I… I'm working on that. If you will give up your career with Viking, we would get you a Green Card so you could join the project. Your knowledge and experience with navigation, especially navigation using the stars, would be an asset to our project. Graduating from the U.S. Merchant Marine Academy is a big plus. The project is an international effort, and we have several on the development team from foreign countries."

"OK, but what would happen when it is time for you to fly off into deep space?"

"On U.S. Navy ships, it is not uncommon to carry non-military advisors among the crew. These advisors are brought on for several reasons, usually involving special knowledge that they possess. You could potentially fill a role on the starship contributing navigational aide and experience to the crew."

"How long would your mission be?"

"We have recently been able to interpret the navigation charts from the UFO captured and stored at Groom Lake to determine that it came from a star system known as Tau Ceti. The system, like our Solar System, comprises eight planets. Two of those planets exist within the Tau Ceti Goldilocks region with gravity and atmosphere similar to Earth. Tau Ceti is approximately twelve light years from Earth."

"So, a round trip mission could take twenty-four years?" asked Ksenia, an expression of shock on her face. "We, or at least I, would be an old woman!"

"Twenty-four years would be at the speed of light. We aren't sure if we could achieve that, so it could be significantly longer. But we are researching faster-than-light speeds that could shorten the trip dramatically."

"I am going to take some time to absorb all of this. We have some life-changing decisions to make, and I want to be comfortable that they will be best for us," said Ksenia.

Chapter Thirty-three

Monday, April 6, 2043, Barnett Mansion

Kristian Barnett sat his desk in his office at Barnett Mansion at 9:55 AM awaiting a briefing from Aaron Adams and Dr. Savannah Richards on the Find Corporation project to develop a smartphone system capable of mind control. During Kristian's and Aaron's trip to the future with The Guardian, they had witnessed a test of a smartphone capable of influencing the mind of a test subject to alter the reality he was seeing regarding the weather. Because of Kristian and Aaron interfering with the test by entering and controlling the mind of the test subject, the test failed twice. The failure resulted in the U.S. Secretary of Defense denouncing the system until a successful test could be presented. Upon return to the year 2042, Kristian successfully started an effort to first become involved in the smartphone project, and then to sabotage the technology behind it.

"Good morning, Savannah, Aaron. Please come in and take a seat," said Kristian, waving his hand at the two leather padded desk chairs facing him. "You've been involved with the Find project for about six months. What do we know?"

"After doing deep dives into the technologies employed by the Russians and Chinese, we are focusing mainly on developments by the Chinese," said Aaron. "They have invested literally trillions of dollars over the past twenty-five years in a plan with four strategies regarding brain science. Brain emulation refers to the development of high-intelligence robots that function like humans. 'Brain control' is the integration of humans with machines into one, allowing soldiers to perform tasks ordinarily impossible to them. This sounds quite similar to our synthetic human program. 'Super brain' involves the use of electromagnetic radiation, such as infrasonic waves or ultrasound, to stimulate human brains and activate the brain's latent potential. The fourth, termed 'controlling the brain,' is about applying advanced technology to interfere with—and manipulate—how people think. This, of course, is precisely what the Find project is attempting to develop."

Aaron continued, "As with most research and development by the Communist Chinese Party (CCP), the Chinese military has, and is, directing their activities. The study into brain science was born out of a vision for how future warfare would develop," Li Peng, a medical researcher at a subsidiary of China's state-run Academy of Military Medical Sciences (AMMS), wrote in an article in 2017. In March 2021, a Chinese military-run newspaper described cloud-powered artificial intelligence (AI) "integrating human and machine" as the key to winning wars. Beijing has spent billions each year since on neuroscience that could draw these scenarios ever closer to reality. Indeed, we have uncovered evidence that shows they have already achieved essentially what Find is attempting to develop."

"The software necessary to effect thought influence is complex but achievable," said Savannah. "I have done some preliminary development with James Handley with Find software development. We have flow charted the primary steps we believe are necessary to deliver altered reality commands to carefully targeted areas of the brain. The key area yet to be determined is the network connectivity necessary to deliver commands generated by the software. Team members from Cyclone and Networks Affiliated are running scenarios through Find AI (Artificial Intelligence) to evaluate all the conditions affecting delivery of the command signals generated by the software."

"What about using Barnett Industries' AI in this effort?" asked Kristian. We've been using AI for two decades to determine the technologies best suited for the delivery of real-time commands across cellular and satellite networks for both military and transportation systems."

"I believe to insert ourselves into that portion of the project, we need to nominate our top scientist for the project," said Aaron.

"Easy choice. KB, setup an appointment as soon as possible with Ragnar Blevins in our Network Development Division and Aaron, Savannah, and me. Ragnar is our chief network and communications scientist and is respected world-wide for his innovative network communications system designs."

The next day, Kristian, Aaron, and Savannah sat down with Ragnar Blevins in Kristian's office at the mansion. "Ragnar, we cannot disclose the specific reasons for our discussion here today. Should your involvement with our activities be recommended, we would need to get your security clearance amended for a highly classified project. Given your existing top secret security clearance, that will not be an issue. We are looking for a means, a technology, that would enable the transmission of commands from a smartphone directly into a specific region of the human brain."

"From what I have researched on this topic, a unique form of low-frequency microwave transmission may fulfill this need. What has not yet been discovered, to my knowledge, is the intensity and frequency of the microwave signal necessary to effect the execution of a command by a human subject. If the intensity is too low, the command may not be received by the subject. If too high, brain damage could result. Many have theorized that experiments regarding microwave transmission into the human brain have been carried out since the beginning of the Twenty-first century. Most noticeably were the odd illnesses experienced by American embassy personnel in Cuba and Moscow. There is speculation that the

Chinese are close to determining the intensity and frequency and may have successfully achieved it. The concern with the Chinese is their known disregard for side effects, including death, that are associated with their experiments on humans. Nothing has been officially reported, but rumors abound."

Kristian and Aaron looked at each other simultaneously, immediately recalling their experience with The Guardian and the Chinese Communist Party virus experiments they witnessed. Death was an expected result of the Caucasian and mixed-race subjects of those experiments.

"Is the challenge to determine and develop the correct technology to deliver commands to the human brain something that Barnett can address?" asked Kristian.

"Definitely," replied Ragnar. "Much research has been conducted determining the best intensities and frequencies for delivering commands to highly critical processors. Our systems controlling autonomous vehicle traffic in large metropolitan areas are but one example. There is also a vast amount of information available regarding the effects of microwave transmission on the human brain. I will engage our AI platform to analyze this data to arrive at the frequencies and intensity that are safe."

"Excellent," said Kristian. "Please work closely with Savannah on this. KB, have Ragnar's security clearance approved for this project. Aaron, please get with Inger Beck at DARPA to introduce Ragnar to the project team."

Chapter Thirty-four

June 9, 2043, Naval Space Command Headquarters, Area 51.

Erik's smartphone buzzed, showing an incoming voice call over a secure frequency. "Commander Richards," he answered.

"Hello Commander, this is Jeremy Winder, project director with DARPA."

"What can I do for you, Mr. Winder?" asked Erik, cautiously.

"Your name was given to me by a Captain Jeffrey… Barnes at Naval Space Command. I understand you are designing and building a starship."

"You are going to have to present me with more credentials than Captain Barnes' name if you expect me to respond to that. How do I know you aren't NCIS (Naval Criminal Investigative Service) or NSA or FBI testing my security compliance?" I have received no verification of your identity from Captain Barnes," said Erik, just as his smartphone buzzed, showing a secure text message had arrived.

"You should receive a secure text or email message from Captain Barnes any moment now," said Jeremy.

"Wait one," said Erik as he looked down at his smartphone.

A message from Captain Barnes read, "Be expecting contact from one Jeremy Winder, DARPA, regarding project."

"OK, Mr. Winder, I have verification from Captain Barnes. What can I do for you?"

"My role at DARPA for the past ten years has been in the development of FTL propulsion for spacecraft. I believe we have information and resources that would be useful to your project."

"FTL, faster-than-light propulsion?" said Erik, astonished at what he was hearing.

"Yes, Commander, faster-than-light propulsion. I would like an opportunity to visit you and your engineering team at Area 51. I have all the necessary clearances to visit you at your new facility.

"S… Sure, Mr. Winder. I can't wait to hear what you guys at DARPA have been up to. When can you come? My team will be available."

"I can be there Thursday, Commander," said Jeremy.

Erik's entire project team was seated in the main conference room at the Space Command's Area 51 headquarters. The conference room featured a large oval glass table surrounded by twenty navy blue leather and chrome swivel chairs. Three large-screen, transparent glass screens in the ceiling could be dropped to eye level for viewing. Each screen could show a visual on both sides of the screen. Holographic images of remote meeting attendees could be accommodated at any seat.

Erik met Jeremy Winder at the facility's front desk. "Mr. Winder, good to meet you," said Erik, extending his hand. "We appreciate you taking the time to brief us on your projects. Please follow me."

"Good afternoon, Commander," said Winder. "I believe your team will be interested in what I am about to speak."

Erik led Winder to the conference room, where introductions proceeded. Erik, standing at the head of the table, said, "Mr. Winder has offered to share DARPA's information compiled over the past ten years regarding faster-than-light travel (FTL)."

Erik then sat down as Winder stood at the head of the table.

"Please call me Jeremy," he started. "As Commander Richards stated, DARPA has had a project in development for about ten years looking at the science behind FTL. Until about 2020, the concept of FTL was considered science fiction. But working with a team of some of the world's best physicists and engineers, we now believe that FTL speeds are achievable."

Winder continued, "In science fiction movies, there are many examples of spaceships racing through space at the speed of light or faster. But is faster-than-light travel possible? In 2021, a research paper written by an American physicist proposed a theory for how faster-than-light travel could be possible. The research was done by Erik Lentz, who did the work at Germany's University of Gottingen. Lentz and his team believed that traveling to distant stars and planets could be possible in the future. But this can happen only if space vehicles travel faster than the speed of light. As you know, light can travel at 299,000 kilometers per second, or approximately six hundred and sixty-nine *hundred million* miles per hour. Physicist Albert Einstein's famous theory of relativity suggests that it is not possible to travel faster than light.

"Dr. Erik Lentz analyzed existing research and discovered gaps in previous 'warp drive' studies. Lentz noticed that there were yet-to-be explored configurations of space-time curvature organized into 'solitons' that have the potential to solve the puzzle while being physically viable. A soliton, in this context, also informally referred to as a warp bubble, is a compact wave that maintains its shape and moves at constant velocity. Lentz derived the Einstein equations for unexplored soliton configurations (where the space-time metric's shift vector components obey a hyperbolic relation), finding that the altered space-time geometries could be formed in a way that worked even with conventional energy sources. The new method uses the very structure of space and time arranged in a soliton to provide a solution to faster-than-light travel, which — unlike other research — would only need sources with positive energy densities. No 'exotic' negative energy densities needed. As a result, the latest research on the subject has centered on theories beyond normal explanations of matter. They call for 'hypothetical particles' and states of matter with unusual physical properties to permit faster-than-light travel. This kind of matter, often referred to as anti-matter, either cannot be found or cannot be manufactured in necessary amounts, the paper states. The new paper places more importance not on theoretical research, but on a possible engineering solution.

"The research describes a plan to permit super fast travel by creating a series of, what the researchers call, solitons to provide the basis for a powerful propulsion system. A soliton is a compact wave that keeps its speed and shape while moving with little loss of energy. The research suggests that such a method could permit travel at any speed.

"The method uses the very structure of space and time arranged in a soliton to provide a solution to faster-than-light travel. Lentz stated that such a 'warp drive' technology could slash travel times. That could make future travel to distant space objects possible.

"The nearest star beyond our solar system is Proxima Centauri. It is about 4.25 light years away. A light year is the distance it takes light to travel in one year. Lentz said that using traditional rocket fuel, it would take about 50,000 to 70,000 years to reach Proxima Centauri. A trip using nuclear fission propulsion technology would take about 100 years, he said. But a light speed trip would take only four years and three months.

"If sufficient energy could be generated, the equations used in this research would allow space travel to Proxima Centauri, our nearest star, and back to Earth in years instead of decades or millennia. That means an individual could travel there and back within their lifetime. In comparison, the current rocket technology would take over 50,000 years for a one-way journey. In addition, the solitons (warp bubbles) could be configured to contain a region with minimal tidal forces, such that the passing of time inside the soliton matches the time outside. This means there would not be the complications of the so-called 'twin paradox' whereby one twin traveling near the speed of light would age much more slowly than the other twin who stayed on Earth. In fact, according to the recent equations, both twins would be the same age when reunited.

"This work has moved the problem of faster-than-light travel one step away from theoretical research in fundamental physics and closer to engineering. The next step is to figure out how to bring down the astronomical amount of energy needed to within the range of today's technologies, such as a large modern nuclear fusion power plant. The researchers' plan promises the hope of faster-than-light-speed travel, which could lead to "distant interstellar travel within a human lifetime." Lentz said a lot of work will be needed to make the method become a reality. To be useful, it would require lowering the energy needed down to the level of modern nuclear fusion power reactors. A way to develop and speed up the solitons must also be created. Lentz saw the research and development process as difficult, but not impossible.

"To summarize, the assumption that the speed of light is the speed limit of the universe has been debunked. Indeed, the alien craft housed here at Area 51 was not brought here under that theory. Here is what we've been able to determine. A series of steps starting with the assumption that velocity (v) must always be less than the speed of light (c) has led to equations that were then used in calculations to prove the original assumption. The Lorentz Transformation (LT) appears in the equation to convert relativistic mass, which is the term that limits velocity to light speed. This is total nonsense. It doesn't prove that v<c; it only assumes it and then forces the assumption via an equation based on that assumption. Here is the logic involved:

1. Einstein postulated that light is the ultimate speed.
2. From this, the LT is derived, and the relativistic energy equation E=mc2 follows from the LT.
3. Scientists then search for evidence to test the postulate.
4. High-energy particles are found.
5. Relativistic energy equation is used to calculate velocity of the particles.
6. The equations prove the postulate that they were based on.

"Basically, the LT has been used to verify itself and the only thing it confirms is that LT=LT. A proof cannot be based on an assumption; it must be based on confirmed facts. If the classical mechanics energy equation had been used instead, an extraordinary speed would have been calculated [4].

"I know this is a lot for some of you to digest. But the bottom line is we now understand the science behind FTL travel. Also, we have the nuclear fusion technology that can provide the power required to achieve FTL.

"What I am suggesting and offering is a partnership with DARPA for developing the FTL engines for your starship. DARPA has been partnering with JPL (Jet Propulsion Laboratories) for several years towards this effort."

Chapter Thirty-five

It is May 2045. Erik and Ksenia have continued their respective careers. Ksenia has been promoted to Chief Navigation Officer (First Officer). Erik remains project manager for the Starship Project, now partnering with the Jet Propulsion Laboratory and DARPA. Erik and Ksenia have maintained their long-distance marriage for two years and both are growing tired of the long periods of separation when Ksenia is on a cruise.

"Erik, when is Ksenia going on leave again?" asked Scarlett. "Isn't she due for a break?"

"Yes, she will arrive at LAX Thursday evening. I'll be taking a few days' leave."

"Will you be staying at the Barnett Center this time?" Kristian has offered one of the Center's guest residences to Erik and Ksenia anytime they want it. Part of the reason is he likes to catch up with Erik regarding any entanglements with The Guardian.

"Yes, Kristian and Ansley have been kind enough to extend their hospitality again. So, I'll be commuting or working from the (Barnett) Center for much of the next three months while Ksenia is on leave."

Friday, May 12, 2045. Erik checked his smartphone for status on

Ksenia's flight from Bergen, Norway. United 432 is now scheduled to arrive at 5:45 PM at the Tom Bradley International Terminal. Erik, on his way to the arrivals hall, stopped and purchased a bouquet of red roses at a gift shop. Soon after, he saw Ksenia exiting the U.S. Customs and Border Patrol, towing her Viking Cruise Lines branded suitcase behind her.

Having not seen each other for three months, they embraced and expressed their love for each other. "I've missed you so much," said Erik. "This last cruise seemed so long."

"I've missed you too," said Ksenia. "The roses are beautiful, thank you. Are we staying at the Center?"

"Yes, we have our bungalow guest house for as long as we need it, per Kristian. Let's go outside and catch an Uber to the mansion."

The autonomous Uber car left the terminal and merged into traffic that was exiting the airport. "What do you feel like having for dinner? I didn't make any plans," said Erik.

"Let's order take out. Something Asian sounds good. That way, we can just relax this evening."

"Sounds great." Erik spoke to Siri: "Siri, find the best rated Asian restaurant in Bel Air and place an order using my and Ksenia's preferences. Setup delivery to the Barnett Center guest cottage for twenty-hundred hours (8 PM). Charge to my credit card on file." Erik always used 24-hour military time with his smartphone.

Arriving at the Barnett Center guest cottage, Erik wheeled Ksenia's bag inside. They then turned and faced each other, touching and kissing lightly at first. As the foreplay became increasingly heated, they moved towards one of the two master bedrooms, dropping their clothes along the way. Once in bed, their passion continued to grow, fueled by their long separation from each other. As he kissed her, first on the lips and then slowly moved down her neck to her breasts and nipples, then down her belly to the light brown patch of hair. They grew more and more excited until he entered her and began carefully thrusting so as not to exert his full cyborg strength on her. After several more minutes, they climaxed together, her moaning and him uttering what sounded like a guttural animal groan. Afterward, he fell off her onto his back. She simply lay there, breathing hard, unable to move.

Just then, they heard a knock on the door of the bungalow. "Oh, it must be the food," said Ksenia, looking at the clock on the dresser across the room that said 8:10 PM in red LED lights.

"We must have been having fun for longer than we thought," said Erik as he leaned over and began kissing her neck.

"Please, get the food," Ksenia squealed.

Erik threw on his boxers and went to the door. As he opened it, he saw the autonomous delivery vehicle rolling down the driveway. The food had been delivered by a delivery bot, programmed to knock when reaching the front door of the residence, set the food down, and return to its vehicle. When the vehicle sensed the door of the residence opening, it left.

Erik carried the food into the kitchen saying, "dinner is served, my dear. I'll open a bottle of wine." The bungalow's wine rack was always stocked with fine wines from the mansion's wine cellar that Kristian selected personally. "Do you want red or white?"

"I'd like white," said Ksenia, exiting the bedroom dressed in an obviously worn t-shirt with "USS Elon Musk" emblazoned on the left breast. The t-shirt hung just above mid-thigh.

"Glad you could dress for dinner," said Erik, laughing.

"It is your shirt! Your boxer shorts are exquisite!" replied Ksenia.

As they began eating, the question that often resulted in tension between them came up again. "Have you given any more thought to us... being together... full time?" asked Erik.

"Erik, you know I want that. It is the one thing I want most. But I am now on the short list for a captaincy. The executive committee that appoints the ship captains is rumored to be interested in naming a woman captain in order to fulfill their perceived need for improving their image as a modern, socially aware corporation. Currently, Viking only has three female captains across both the ocean and river cruises."

"I know that becoming a ship's captain is your lifelong career goal. But, what about us... our goals for us? The cruises, the separations are becoming more difficult to endure. We were wrong in thinking they'd become more routine. If you are named a captain, it would likely mean years before we would finally settle down."

"What about you, Erik?" started Ksenia, her accent becoming more pronounced, showing she was becoming emotionally aroused. "In what, two or three years, will you be leaving on a years-long journey to the stars? If I'm a housewife at that point, what am I supposed to do? You could be gone for a decade or longer while I grow old and gray by myself."

"I need to bring you with me or resign from the project," said Erik. "I will not leave you for years at a time. But I need you to be open-minded regarding how we can do that. I believe you have skills from your education and years at sea, especially with navigation, to be an asset to the project."

"I will always listen to your ideas and suggestions. Just know that my career is very important to me, as yours is to you."

They finished their meal, cleaned up afterwards, and sat on the leather sofa in front of the holographic TV. They watched an old Star Trek movie featuring Chris Pine as Captain Kirk. Erik had seen the movie a dozen times and still loved it. Finishing their bottle of wine, both fell asleep before the movie concluded.

The next morning, they awoke at sunrise. "I think I'd like to go for a run," said Ksenia. "I don't get many opportunities to run while I'm at sea. Occasionally, around the deck is all I get."

Just then Erik's smartphone buzzed, showing an incoming call on the secure government line. "Commander Richards," he answered.

"Erik, Jeffrey Barnes. I need to send you a top-secret portfolio of documents for your immediate response. Do you have your laptop with you?

"Yes, sir. Ready and waiting, Captain."

"Good. The portfolio is on its way. Please confirm when you receive it."

Erik checked his secure email on his smartphone and saw the email from Captain Barnes. "Yes, sir, I have the portfolio and will begin reviewing it immediately.

"I guess I'll have to go on my run alone," said Ksenia.

"Yeah, sorry, love. Even though I'm technically on leave, I'm really never on leave," said Erik.

Ksenia left the bungalow and ran past Barnett Center, down the winding driveway to the crossing boulevard. She turned right and crossed the boulevard so she would face traffic. After another half mile, she turned left on a narrow side street. As she ran, she admired the extravagant estates with their perfectly manicured gardens and lawns. She crested a steep hill and saw a large panel truck coming towards her at a high rate of speed. She moved as close to the edge of the pavement as she could without falling in the drainage ditch to her left. As she continued to run, she kept her focus, looking down on the road's edge. The right bumper of the truck bashed her on her right side, resulting in multiple fractures of her right leg, pelvis, arm, wrist, and shoulder. Several of her ribs on the right side of her body were fractured and one rib punctured a lung. She spun around to her right, fracturing her neck, and fell, unconscious, into the ditch.

The driver of the truck slammed on the brakes. The man riding shotgun said with panic in his voice, "what the hell? Did you just hit that girl?"

"I… I don't know. Get out and look!"

The passenger stepped down out of the truck and walked to the back of the truck, looking in the drainage ditch, when he saw a body that appeared to be that of a woman lying face down about ten yards up the hill. He stepped into the ditch and grabbed her shoulder to turn her face up. He heard a moan. "Call 911!" he yelled. "There's a woman hurt here in the ditch!"

Chapter Thirty-six

Erik opened the portfolio sent by Captain Barnes. It started with the usual headings placed on top-secret documents: FOR YOUR EYES ONLY. As he read the document, his thoughts immediately returned to the experience he had with The Guardian and the incidents in China in 2028 with the Chinese Communist Party's racially targeted, deadly virus. He recalled that there had never been any mention of the virus in the news media or reference to the Chinese laboratory that had been mysteriously destroyed shortly following the incident with The Guardian.

According to the document he was reading, evidence has surfaced that points to a U.S. secret space fleet. Its program is named "Solar Warden" and has a large space station and space docking facility, and forty-three small scout ships. The space station was constructed in the early 1990s to house the growing number of scout ships.

The U.S. Space Fleet operated under the U.S. Naval Space Command (NSC), headquartered in Dahlgren, Virginia. There are approximately 300 personnel at the NSC Dahlgren facility. The U.S. Space Fleet's vessels are staffed by Naval Space Cadre officers, whose training has earned them the prestigious 6206-P Space Operations specialty designation, after they have graduated from advanced education at the Naval Postgraduate School in Monterey,

California and earned a Master of Science degree in Space Systems Operations. Erik possesses these same credentials and Scarlett will attend this school soon. Both the Navy and the Marine Corps furnish men and women officers to this program.

The purpose of the Space Fleet is to monitor the activities of potential subversives and terrorists on Earth, and to police those activities with force as necessary. Additionally, the Fleet is to surveil any potential threats to earth from extraterrestrial sources.

After about an hour of reading through the materials, Erik got up and went into the kitchen to fix a cup of coffee. As he was pouring the coffee, his smartphone buzzed, showing a call labeled as "911" flashed on his screen. The call did not come in on his secure Pentagon line.

"Is this Erik Richards?" the caller said without introducing herself.

"Y… Yes, who are you?"

"I am officer Rachel Gonzales with the Los Angeles County Sheriff's Department. Do you know a Ksenia Richards?"

"Yes, yes, she is my wife! Is she in trouble?"

"Ms. Richards has been critically injured in a motor vehicle accident. She was transported by air ambulance to Bel Air Memorial Hospital. If you give me your location, I will pick you up and take you to the hospital. Ms. Richards is in very serious condition."

Erik quickly threw on shorts, a t shirt, and some athletic shoes. Officer Gonzales was in front of the Center bungalow in less than ten minutes. "Mr. Richards, sorry to meet you under these circumstances. Please buckle up. We are going airborne to get you to the hospital as quickly as possible."

The flying police car's short wings extended from their folded position against the two doors and nacelles containing the craft's motors unfolded and turned vertically. Officer Gonzales spoke to the vehicle's AI. "Bel Air Memorial Hospital." The engines cycled up, and the car rose vertically. Once reaching the pre-programmed altitude, the nacelles pitched forward and quickly sped up the craft to ninety miles per hour. The car's AI said, "ETA four minutes."

"What… What happened to Ksenia?" asked Erik, his panic evident in his voice.

"Apparently she was jogging on a narrow street without sidewalks when an approaching truck struck her. Her injuries are quite extensive, and she needs immediate surgery. The hospital requires approval of next of kin for the surgery."

The craft landed on the hospital's helipad on the roof of the facility. A hospital employee walked up to Erik as he stepped out of the police vehicle. "Mr. Richards, I am Marsha Peters, a social worker for the hospital. Please follow me."

"How's Ksenia?" Erik asked as they walked to the door to the elevators.

"She's in surgery now," said Peters. "I understand you are her husband. We need you to sign her authorization for treatment. We'll go to my office and complete that as quickly as possible. Then you can go to the surgical waiting room, where doctors will update you as soon as they are able."

As soon as Erik got to the surgery waiting area, he sent a 911 text to Savannah, Kristian, Ansley, and Aaron that said, "Ksenia badly injured. In surgery at Bel Air." He then ordered Siri to contact Ksenia's parents, Carl and Ebba, and get them on the phone. A few moments later, his smartphone buzzed, showing an incoming call.

"Carl, Ebba?" said Erik.

"We are both here," said Carl. "What has happened?"

"Ksenia has been in an accident and is seriously injured. She is in surgery now at Bel Air Memorial Hospital. If you are able, one or both of you should come to Los Angeles as soon as possible."

After a few moments of silence, Carl said, "What happened?" Erik then repeated what Officer Gonzales had told him regarding the accident. "My God!" said Carl. "We will be on the next plane to Los Angeles. But the only way to do that is to depart Bergen Airport, hours away from us."

"I will have my travel service get a flying car to your estate as quickly as possible to take you to Bergen," said Erik. "Don't worry about accommodations in LA. You can stay at the Barnett Center guest house with me as long as you need to."

Erik then called Captain Barnes on his secure line. "Captain Barnes," said Barnes, picking up his smartphone. The speakerphone was automatically deactivated when calls coming in on the secure line were answered, requiring that the phone be picked up.

"Captain, Erik. I have some bad news. Ksenia has been in an accident and is in critical condition. She is in surgery now."

"Erik, I'm very sorry to hear that. Please let me know if there is anything you need us to do."

"I had time to review the materials you sent this morning. I'll get back to that as soon as I'm able. Very interesting information."

"Erik, no hurry about that. It can wait until Ksenia is stable and recovering."

"Thanks, Captain."

Thirty minutes later, Savannah, Aaron, and Ansley appeared in the waiting room. Savannah spoke first as she hugged Erik. "Erik, what happened? How is Ksenia?

"She apparently was hit by a truck while jogging this morning. That's about all I know so far. She is still in surgery. I haven't spoken to any of the doctors treating her yet. Hopefully, I'll get a status soon."

"Were you with her when she was hit?" asked Savannah.

"No, and I feel terrible that I wasn't. Just before we were to go out for a run, I received a communication from my CO that he was sending some material he needed me to review right away. So, I told Ksenia to go ahead without me. The next thing I know, a sheriff's deputy was calling to tell me Ksenia's been in an accident. The deputy picked me up at the Center and flew me straight to the hospital. If I had gone with her, maybe this whole thing might have been avoided," Erik said, tears forming in his eyes. Later, he recalled being amazed at how his synthetic body could emulate a human body's response in emotional situations.

"You can't say that," said Ansley. "Please don't blame yourself, Erik. This was not your fault."

Chapter Thirty-seven

Another hour passed when a woman dressed in surgical scrubs walked into the waiting room and said, "Erik Richards?"

Erik nearly jumped up from his seat and stepped in front of the Woman, "yes, I am Erik Richards." Savannah, Ansley, and Aaron gathered around the woman and Erik.

"I am Doctor Kristen Conkling, surgeon on your wife's case. Ksenia is still in surgery, but I wanted you to know that we believe she will survive. Fortunately, she had no damage to her skull and there was no clear physical brain damage. She did, however, suffer extensive orthopedic damage, including extensive damage to the thoracic region of her spine, as well as losing her spleen and right lung. Her neck was fractured, which may cause partial or full paralysis. Her right arm could not be saved and has been amputated just below the elbow. Also, her right shoulder was shattered. The surgery she is undergoing now is, in part, to reconstruct her shoulder. Do you have any questions?"

Erik stood silent, staring at Doctor Conkling for several moments. "Will she be able to walk again?"

"In my experience, the level of damage to her spine would prevent that, at least without stem cell and/or chemical intervention. But the damage to the entire right side of her body, where she was struck by the vehicle, may negate any advantage gained through spinal restoration."

"But she will live?"

"Barring any setback, yes, she will survive."

Erik's smartphone buzzed, showing an incoming call on his personal line. "Hello, this is Erik."

"Erik, Kristian here. I am so sorry to hear about Ksenia's accident. Have you received any updates from the doctors?"

"Yes, just a few minutes ago, a Dr. Conkling told us that Ksenia is expected to survive the accident. But a full recovery is unlikely. She had extensive damage to her spine and the entire right side of her body. Her neck was broken, and she may be paralyzed. Her right arm was amputated. They are still operating, reconstructing her shoulder," said Erik, his emotion clear in his voice.

"My God! How terrible. I am sorry that I can't be there with you, but you know the reason. In the meantime, if there is anything I can do, anything, please ask. You have the full resources of Barnett Industries at your disposal. Please keep me informed of Ksenia's progress."

"Thank you, Kristian. I really appreciate all you've done for Ksenia and me."

As the days passed, Ksenia was maintained in an induced coma to keep her out of pain and to enable her body to heal. Carl and Ebba had arrived late the day after Ksenia's surgery and finally persuaded Erik to get some rest. Erik had stayed by her side day and night since the accident.

After day five, Erik knew he had to return to the bungalow to recharge his body's batteries and try to rest his mind. But he found it difficult, if not impossible, to quiet his mind, thinking of Ksenia, her recovery, and their future, which had been completely changed forever. He returned to the material sent by Captain Barnes to get his mind off of Ksenia for a brief time.

Continuing to read through material, Erik found that many of the UFO/UAP encounters reported since the early years of the century were the craft used by Solar Warden. That explained the propensity of the sightings to have occurred near military ships and aircraft, as well as near nuclear facilities. Erik then found a reference to the Chinese Communist Party laboratory destroyed by Solar Warden. The document stated the lab was destroyed for developing extinction-level pathogens. The destruction resulted from targeting the lab with an orbital-based energy beam.

Erik picked up his smartphone and dialed Captain Barnes on a secure line.

"Barnes," was the response.

"Captain, Erik. I've just read over the material you sent. The United States has a well-established base of tactical spacecraft patrolling the planet?"

"Yes. I first became aware or Solar Warden a few months ago. I have been working to find out the implications for our starship project. Solar Warden does not have the technology to support deep space travel. It is strictly a planetary observation force. But they possess highly advanced weaponry. The only action they have taken is the destruction of the Chinese lab. Solar Warden has yet to be detected by any other nation, including the Chinese. The base station shielding that scrambles satellite and photo detection has been very effective.

"The commander of Solar Warden is a Captain William Sims. Captain Sims has offered, with authorization from SecDef, to engage with our starship project team to exchange information beneficial to both commands. I will send you Captain Sims' contact information. Please contact him at your earliest to arrange a meeting.

"How is Ksenia doing?"

"Her recovery will be long and difficult. According to her doctors, she will probably never regain full functionality. Right now, she remains non-responsive to stimulation below her waist. She will be kept in an induced coma for at least several more days."

"Please know that we are ready and willing to help in any way we can."

"Thanks, Captain."

Chapter Thirty-eight

Kristian was sitting at his desk in his office at the mansion when he received a call from Savannah. "Kristian, I have some exciting news regarding our search for a cure for ALS. May I come up to your office to explain?"

"Yes, by all means. Please come right away."

Savannah entered Kristian's office a few minutes later. "Good morning, Savannah. Please come in and take a seat."

"Kristian, I believe we have found a cure for ALS. Ansley has been working with a newly developed nanobot that is adaptable in many situations. Her first application is to incorporate the bots into the synthetic skin of a cyborg to act as batteries that charge using ambient light. My group has been working with the bots to use them to restore nerve and muscle control destroyed by ALS. We have been working with several volunteers afflicted with ALS to test the effectiveness of the bots in restoring functionality. We started with extremities of the test subjects and saw an immediate improvement in motion control of fingers, hands, and arms. Two of our volunteers have been able to stand without help leaning only on a physical therapy walking bar. One of our test subjects was probably only weeks away from death. We injected the bots into his heart, lungs, and throat. Within hours, we saw improved breathing and oxygen saturation. He can now speak and swallow soft foods. Not only does this technology block the progression of the disease, but it also effectively reverses the damage caused."

"Savannah, that is absolutely amazing! I knew Ansley was working with nano technology to improve her synthetics. But I didn't realize that you were working with the same technology. How are the bots powered and how long will they be functional once introduced to the body?"

"Actually, the bots we use are partially human tissue. Placental stem cells are incorporated into the bot's architecture. The bots are powered by the human body itself. We expect the bots to live as long as the body lives. In contrast, the nanobots Ansley is using are powered by energy, either from light or through artificial charging done routinely today by... the cyborgs."

"When will you be ready to go public on your discovery?"

"Soon, I hope. I would like to show a patient that has completely recovered from a documented case of ALS before going public. Of course, going public will require FDA approval for the treatment. Phase 1 through Phase 3 clinical trials normally take several years to complete. But given the success we have seen as well as the importance of a successful treatment regimen to those afflicted with ALS, I will apply for an emergency use authorization, EUA, to bypass Phase 1 and 2 trials and go directly to Phase 3 human trials."

"It sounds like I may finally return to public life," said Kristian, his voice reflecting his excitement at the prospect.

"I have additional news regarding the nanobots. Since they are programmable, they should be able to be used for the Find Corporation mind control project, or as it is now dubbed, *MildMeld*. The nanobots theoretically can be programmed to target areas of the brain, synapses, where perception is formed and decisions are made. Upon receiving commands from a specified source, they activate and cause the brain to see altered reality, accept altered truths, and act on these perceptions or carry out specific commands."

"How will the nanobots be introduced into the brains of millions of targeted individuals?" asked Kristian.

"Again, still theory, but the thinking is that they could be introduced as a virus capable of breaking through the human blood-brain barrier. In order to distribute a viable smartphone capable of accepting and transmitting information to the nanobots, Find and the two partnering telecommunications companies would offer a free, highly advanced smartphone for enrolling in steeply discounted cellular services. The smartphone would carry a harmless vector, or virus, that would infect the user upon first touch as they opened the package containing the phone. The project team believes enough subjects could be infected with the nanobots in less than one year to cause major changes aligned with the political will of those controlling the political narrative."

"Would we have a way to counter, or sabotage, the messages being generated?"

"That is the beauty of this technology. Unbeknownst to the controlling entity, we could establish a way to disable the nanobots or introduce alternate messages using the same delivery system. The smartphones would have two separate microprocessors. One that would provide normal, expected smartphone functionality under the most common operating systems in use, iOS and Android. The second processor, created in a virtual session under the main processor, would provide the ability to receive commands from an approved, cloud-based source and relay the commands to the nanobots in the subject's brain using low-frequency, harmless microwaves."

"Savannah, this sounds more like science fiction than fact. What do you expect the timeline to be for the development of this project?"

"If I were to estimate how long it will take to get to a functioning demonstration of the technology, I would say a minimum of three to five years."

"Interesting. That could put it right on the timeline The Guardian showed us when we traveled to the year 2052. Please continue your efforts, Savannah. This is fantastic news!"

Chapter Thirty-nine

August 2045

Erik, Savannah, and Ansley entered Ksenia's room at Bel Air Hospital. Ksenia had been aroused after five weeks in the induced coma in late June. Erik, as well as Ksenia's parents, Carl and Ebba, had spent as much time as possible with Ksenia since she had awakened. For Ksenia, depression was as much an affliction as was her physical condition. She remained paralyzed below the waist and the prognosis was that she would never walk again, that her spine was too damaged to undergo a restoration procedure.

"Good morning, love," said Erik. "I've brought a couple of visitors with me today. They would like to talk to you about an opportunity to recover from the accident."

"Oh?" said Ksenia. Her depression had resulted in her Scandinavian accent becoming more pronounced.

"Hello, Ksenia," said Ansley. "What if we could fully restore you to complete health? Would that interest you?"

"H… How would you do that?" asked Ksenia, her voice trembling with emotion.

"You know, of course, that we restored Erik to full health after his accident in space. If you are interested in transitioning to a synthetic body, we may do the same for you. Now to do that, Erik, Savannah, and I would have to make a case for the transition to the Department of Defense. But we may just have enough justification, as well as people in the right positions, to achieve approval. So, the question is, would you want us to proceed with obtaining approval to transition you to a synthetic body?"

After a few silent moments, with tears forming in her eyes, Ksenia said, "I would give anything to have my life back. But how could you justify this to the U.S. military? I am not even a citizen of this country."

"My plan would be to present the case that we need a member on my project team with your education, skills and experience," said Erik. "Your navigational skills are outstanding. Further, as a synthetic, you would make a perfect crew, er, team member on the project. In addition, Savannah and I would enlist the support of our uncle, Senator Richards, who is highly influential on the Senate Armed Services Committee. I will put my life and career on the line to enable you to realize your dreams, Ksenia, and will pull out all the stops to do so." Erik realized he'd almost inadvertently spilled the beans about the starship project in front of Ansley and Savannah.

"Returning to a full life would be a miracle. I will do anything to realize that miracle," said Ksenia as tears ran down her cheeks.

Later that morning, Erik called Captain Barnes on his secure encrypted line. "Good morning, sir. Erik Richards here. I have a matter of the utmost importance to discuss with you. Is this a good time?"

"Yes, Commander. Please continue," said Barnes.

"You know that Ksenia's prognosis is poor, and she is not expected to walk again. Fortunately, however, she experienced no head or brain trauma from the accident. So, I would like to submit her for consideration for transition to a synthetic body."

"Whoa… whoa, stop right there, Commander. While I can fully understand your desire to give her back her life, she is not in the military. She isn't even a citizen, is she?"

"Sir, no, she is not a citizen. But please hear me out. Ksenia is an inactive member of the Norwegian Royal Navy. She graduated from the United States Merchant Marine Academy. She has been employed as a first officer for Viking Cruise Lines with primary responsibility for ship operations and navigation. I believe she would be an excellent candidate for the starship project, given her navigational expertise. Finally, I believe she would be an excellent candidate for the crew should she transition to a synthetic."

"Commander, I am sure we have U.S. citizens, even naval officers, who would equal or better Ksenia's navigational skills. So, tell me how I can justify your recommendation to Command."

"You are probably right, Captain. We undoubtedly have people qualified from within our own country. The problem is that they are not synthetic. The decision has been made that it will be a top priority for the crew of the starship to comprise synthetics, cyborgs. Currently, we have only Scarlett and me that qualify. To prepare an unknown candidate for both the project and planned space travel will take several months. Ksenia could be ready for active duty within nine months, which would allow us to meet our timeline for launch. Waiting for another qualified synthetic would undoubtedly delay the launch phase of the project."

"You make a compelling argument, Erik. Please draft your request and address it to me. I will present it to Command. But know that it is a stretch and unlikely to be approved."

"Thank you, sir. That is all I can ask."

Chapter Forty

Erik returned to the guest house from the hospital after staying by Ksenia's side while she slept most hours of the day. Ksenia's parents, Carl and Ebba, had given Erik the opportunity for Erik to recharge his synthetic body's batteries. He quickly undressed and connected the charging and data storage cable to the connector located under a flap of artificial skin at the back of his neck. As he lay down, he attempted to start the mental exercises given to the cyborgs to relax his mind. Although the synthetic body required no sleep, the human mind of the synthetic required periodic rest. But thoughts of Ksenia's condition, her recovery, their future were followed by how patient the Navy would regard him splitting his time between the starship project and Ksenia. After what seemed like hours, Erik could finally relax his mind and enter a state between actual sleep and wakefulness that enabled his mind to rest, dream, and recharge.

After an indeterminate amount of time, Erik sensed someone else's presence in his bedroom. "Who's there?" he said, as he opened his mind's eyes. Then he realized who was there. "Guardian?"

"Yes, Erik. I have come because we have work," said The Guardian, who now stood before Erik, whose spirit was now fully awake and separated from his synthetic body, dressed in his usual outfit of t-shirt, jeans, a long leather coat, cowboy boots and a Stetson.

"Guardian, given the serious situation with Ksenia, am I your best choice for an assignment now?"

"Erik, yes, you are the most qualified of the spirits for this assignment. You have a military background, which you will see is needed."

"Scarlett has a military background as well. Could she fill the role you envision?"

"During the time in history that we will address, women do not have the influence to be successful with what you are about to do. Also, recall that after completing your assignment, you will be brought back into this time at exactly the point you departed. There will be no effect on your current situation with Ksenia. Here, take my arm and we will go where we are needed."

Erik immediately finds himself standing in Thomas Jefferson's house, at Oak Hill, Virginia, which Jefferson had abandoned facing capture by the British. He and The Guardian observed two men who appear to be high-ranking British military offers discussing what appears to be war strategy. "Guardian, where… when are we?"

"We are in 1781, nearing the conclusion of the Revolutionary War of the United States. The two men before you are Generals Benedict Arnold and Charles Cornwallis. Listen, as this discussion has profound information relative to the outcome of the war."

"I'm telling you, General Cornwallis, you need to establish your headquarters far from the coast. On the coast, you are more vulnerable to attack by the armies of the Colonies and the French, supported by the French Navy."

"I will take your advice under advisement, Benedict," replied Cornwallis gruffly. Cornwallis had a low opinion of Arnold whom he considered a traitor even though he abandoned the Continental Army for the British. Cornwallis did not favor taking advice from a traitor.

"In August 1781 Cornwallis established his base at a small village on the Virginia coast, Yorktown," said The Guardian.

"Yorktown. Cornwallis surrendered to George Washington at Yorktown, setting the stage for ending the war," said Erik.

Erik and The Guardian are then instantly transported to a home in the Dobbs Ferry section of Greenburg, New York, owned by Joseph Appleby, a 2nd lieutenant in the First Regiment of Westchester County, New York Militia. Appleby had opened his home to be the headquarters of George Washington's Continental Army.

"George Washington has been planning to attack the British at New York City for at least two months," said The Guardian. "Washington believes that his chances of successfully expelling the British are by attacking them there. Washington also carries a desire for revenge for the manner in which his army was expelled from New York earlier in the war. The commander of the French Army, General Jean Baptiste Donatien de Vimeur, comte de Rochambeau, was not keen on attacking the British at New York City. He preferred Admiral DeGrasse of the French Navy sail up the Chesapeake Bay and attack the British on the coast of Virginia. Erik, your assignment will be to persuade General Washington to heed the advice of General Rochambeau and march to the south."

"So, I am to take control of the mind of the father of our country and force him to make a decision he doesn't believe in?" said Erik somewhat emotionally.

"Enter his mind, yes. Take control, no," said The Guardian. "You will enter Washington's mind while he is sleeping and appear to him in a dream. You will appear to him in your full-dress naval uniform and introduce yourself as a United States naval officer from the future. You will then tell him he will end the war by defeating Cornwallis at Yorktown. To aide his success, he must write an open letter to General Marquis de La Fayette that details plans for attacking the British at New York. The letter must be open text and mailed via normal post, enabling the British to capture it."

"This certainly sounds different from the missions I've had with you previously," said Erik.

"Yes, but we must allow Washington to make his own decision regarding the change of strategy to march to Yorktown. If you made it for him, he would doubt his own cognizance."

"I... I've not done this... dream thing before. Will this really work?"

"A person's dreams are their own and no one else need know of them. You will appear to him to be much more real than in a dream that his own mind fabricates."

Late in the evening, General Washington prepared for bed, removing his uniform and boots, and donning his sleeping gown. Although he was near exhaustion, he could not fall asleep immediately. He weighed the pros and cons of his strategy to attack the British at New York, reinforcing his belief that New York was the place to expel the British. Exhaustion finally overcame his heightened mental state, and he drifted into a deep sleep.

"Erik, Washington is now in a deep sleep. Now Is the Time to enter his mind."

Erik hesitated for a moment before he entered the general's mind. "General Washington," he started. Erik saw the General's spirit rise from the sleeping body.

"W... Who are you? What are you doing here? What do you want with me?" said Washington. "What is that uniform you are wearing?"

"Sir, I am an officer in the United States Navy, two hundred sixty years in the future. I have come to give you insight into how you must proceed in order to win the war."

"I must be dreaming," said Washington. "This is just my mind still dealing with the advice of others, including General Rochambeau, trying to convince me to march to the south, to Virginia."

"Does this really feel like a dream, General?" said Erik, pointing at Washington's sleeping body.

"I must be dreaming," Washington said, as his spirit turned to look down at himself sleeping.

"But this dream..., this vision, is real, General. If you fail to follow my advice, you risk losing the war."

"How do I know what you say is real? How am I to trust a vision?"

"Think about it, General. I am from a time two hundred sixty years in the future when the United States, the country you are fighting for, is the most powerful nation in the world. In that time, you are referred to as the father of our nation. If you believe in that future, you must believe me."

"Then, just how am I to win the war, spirit?"

"You must march to the south instead of attacking New York. The French navy is sailing for the Chesapeake Bay and will block the British Navy from defending Cornwallis at Yorktown. You will defeat Cornwallis and bring about an end to the war."

"Hmm… that is what General Rochambeau has been telling me. I will have to take this under advisement."

"There is another action you must take for you to succeed. You must write a communique, in plain text stating plans for attacking New York, to the Marquis de Lafayette, based in Virginia and observing General Cornwallis' movements. Send the communique by normal post. This will enable the British to capture it and force preparation for an attack by your army at New York. This communique will prevent General Henry Clinton from sending reinforcements to Cornwallis in Virginia."

Erik left Washington's mind and returned to The Guardian. "Guardian, what would have happened had Washington stubbornly refused to march to the south and defeat Cornwallis at Yorktown?"

"The Continental Army would have experienced defeat at New York and, ultimately, would have lost the War of Independence to the British. This would have transformed history, not only for the United States but also the rest of the world. In the end, Evil would have gained control of humanity, which would have been subjugated to tyranny and slavery."

Erik's spirit was instantly reunited with his synthetic body where he lay in awe regarding what he had experienced. The United States was so close to failure during the Revolution, and he had just played a role in saving the country at its very beginning.

Chapter Forty One

September 2045

Erik was in his office at the Area 51 complex where his team was developing the plans for Earth's first starship when his smartphone showed an incoming call on his secure line. He picked up the phone and said, "Richards."

"Erik, Jeff Barnes. I have some news on you request regarding Ksenia. The decision is to permit Ksenia's transition to a synthetic body. However, federal funds cannot be used for the transition. In addition, the cost of time spent by federal employees or contractors on the transition may not be billed to the federal government. The decision to prohibit the use of federal funds is subject to reconsideration in the future, depending on Ksenia's application for U.S. citizenship and her actual employment by Navy Space Command on your project."

Erik was silent for a few moments, then said with emotion in his voice, "The cost of a transition is well into eight figures and approaches the cost of a brand-new small jet aircraft. H… How are we supposed to pay that?"

"Erik, frankly, I am surprised that the decision came down

in your favor. Knowing SecDef's negative opinions regarding the synthetics program, I feel there must have been influence from other sources in your favor. If I were you, I'd take the decision as it is and look for funding to carry out your plans."

"I understand, sir. Thank you for your help in this matter. I know it cannot have been easy," said Erik.

"Good luck, Commander," said Captain Barnes. "I sincerely hope things work out for you and Ksenia."

Erik then had his digital assistant setup a conference call with Ansley and Savannah to relay the terms of the decision that he had just received. A few hours later, the three of them joined the call. Erik relayed the terms. After several moments of silence, Savannah said, "I… I guess that is positive news, Erik. At least there is hope that we can transition Ksenia without interference from the federal government."

Erik, still somewhat emotional, replied, "But how in the hell am I supposed to come up with the tens of millions of dollars needed for the transition? Ansley, what do you estimate the costs would be?"

"You're not far off regarding the cost. Even donating my time and Barnett's medical facilities, we're still looking at a cost north of fifty million dollars."

"Thanks, both of you, for your support in this matter. I will explain the situation to Ksenia when I return to LA on Friday."

Later that evening, Erik's smartphone showed an incoming call from Kristian Barnett. "Hello, Kristian. What can I do for you?" answered Erik.

"Erik, Ansley just explained the response you received from the federal government regarding Ksenia. I am calling to let you know that Ansley and I will use our personal resources to fund Ksenia's transition to a synthetic body.

"K… Kristian, the costs for this are enormous! You must know it is highly doubtful that we could ever repay you."

"Not true, Erik. Your plans for Ksenia, should she transition, is to bring her under your naval command in a special role. If she becomes a U.S. citizen and is successful in the role you envision for her, the decision regarding funding by the federal government can be reconsidered. Ansley and I are confident that you and Ksenia will be successful with your plans."

"Kristian, you know that the federal government reversing the decision on funding Ksenia's transition is remote."

"I am an entrepreneur. Taking risks is what I do, and I will take a risk on Ksenia and you. Frankly, we are confident that you will be successful."

"Kristian, I don't know what to say. I am speechless. How can we thank you?" said Erik, emotion clear in his voice.

"You can thank us by being successful, Erik."

"I would like to give Ksenia the news when I return to LA tomorrow evening. Would you and Ansley be available to meet us at the guest house around 7 PM?"

"I believe so, but I will check with Ansley. If you don't hear from me before then, we'll see you at the guest house."

A few minutes past 7 PM Friday, the doorbell at the Barnett Center guest house rang. Erik answered the door. "Ansley, Kristian, thank you for coming. I've not told Ksenia of the decision from Washington to let her transition or of your amazing offer. I thought we'd tell her together."

Ksenia was sitting in her highly specialized wheelchair she controlled with her mind. "Kristian, Ansley, how nice to see you," said Ksenia as they entered her room. "What brings you here now?"

"Ksenia, we have some news we believe you will like," said Erik. "The government has approved your transition to a synthetic body."

Ksenia raised her good hand to her mouth as tears formed in her eyes. "I am… speechless. I don't know what to say."

"There is one caveat that came with the approval," continued Erik. "The government will not pay for the transition."

"What does that mean?" replied Ksenia. "These… transitions must cost millions of dollars. How will we ever get the funds?"

"Kristian, Ansley?" said Erik.

"Ksenia, Ansley and I have decided to fund your transition

with one condition. Once you have regained full functionality in a synthetic body, you will pursue U.S. citizenship and join Erik's project with the Navy," said Kristian.

"Ksenia, while the government will not pay for the transition now, that decision may be reconsidered when you can show incontrovertible proof that you are an asset to the United States," said Erik. "As I've told you many times, your education and experience make you a likely fit with my Navy project."

"Kristian, Ansley, your offer is incredible. I will be happy to do what is necessary to repay you. You are giving me my life back. Trying to repay you is the least I can do," said Ansley.

Chapter Forty-two

Project leads took their seats in the SpaceCom conference room at Area 51 in response to a status meeting called by Erik. In attendance were Commander Erik Richards (program director), Scarlett Bross (starship pilot), System Engineering Manager Rick Williams, Deputy Engineering Manager Kirk Banner, Chief Engineer, Adam Stanner, Deputy Chief Engineer Keith Callahan Deputy Chief Engineer Soren Amakov, and Flight Systems Manager Raymond Billings.

"Good morning, gentlemen… and lady," began Erik, nodding at Scarlett. As you know, we are nearing the three-year mark in our project and will soon begin the construction phase. One thing that means is that we will spend much of our time overseeing the construction. What has changed from our original concept of constructing and assembling the ship entirely in orbit, is we will construct most of the parts and some of the ship's sections here at Area 51. Parts will then be shuttled to the base station for the assembly phase. So, while you will still see frequent trips to the base station, you will spend much of your time right here.

"Regarding Ksenia, she is recuperating at the Barnett Center for Neurological Restoration in Bel Air, where she will soon undergo surgeries and procedures that are expected to result in a full recovery from her injuries. Her prognosis has improved significantly because of methods pioneered by Barnett Center."

"That is incredible news," said Scarlett. "I am sitting here today thanks to Barnett Center."

"Rick, what is the status regarding the development of the nuclear fusion engines?"

"The prototype engine is undergoing tests at JPL. So far, a few needed modifications have been identified and are under development. The engine portion of the project remains on track," said Rick Williams.

"Any of the modifications critical to the engine design?" asked Erik.

"No, the design remains solid. The modifications mostly address some weaknesses found in the engine's durability to withstand the high temperatures and radiation shield generated during nuclear fusion. Design AI is being used for the corrections."

"What do we know regarding the development of the space warp bubble?"

"I have been working almost exclusively with Dr. Jeremy Winder from DARPA," said Keith Callahan. "Nearly everything associated with the underlying technology of the Lentz Drive Bubble remains mostly theoretical. We have conducted tests that have proven the concept on a small scale where we have been able to accelerate small particles encapsulated in a soliton to many times light speed using the Lentz drive technology. The speed of the particles is measured using a receiver of the particles on Mars. At the speed of light, approximately 186,000 miles per second, the particles would take two-hundred fifteen seconds to reach Mars. The particles reached Mars in a little over two seconds, indicating a speed nearly ten times the speed of light. At a minimum, if we can employ Lentz technology by encapsulating communications in a Lentz warp bubble, we could eliminate the current lag in communications between Earth and Mars."

"Do we still think that this technology will enable FTL speed for our ship?" *Warp factor 9, Scotty!*

"Too early to confirm, but it appears things are still heading for a positive outcome," said Keith.

"I have another, rather startling item to share with you," continued Erik. Looking sternly at each of the team members directly in their eyes, "this item carries the highest confidentiality and must not be discussed outside of this room. There is a secret base in orbit where a group that goes by the name of *Solar Warden* whose primary mission is to watch for alien spacecraft. They also observe, and have reacted in the past, to events perpetrated by Earth's governments that threaten the planet and/or humanity. The spacecraft they employ are based on and are very similar to the alien craft that crashed in Roswell, New Mexico in 1947. And they carry the most advanced weapons yet deployed, as well as the ability to cloak the spacecraft from both radar and visibility.

"The base is hidden using advanced arrays of cameras and energy shielding like that which hides the Roswell spacecraft hangar and laboratory here at Area 51. We will employ this technology to hide our orbital construction facilities. I will contact the commander of Solar Warden after this meeting to arrange a tour for those of us involved with the operation of the construction facility."

The room fell silent for what seemed like several minutes. *Did they comprehend what I just told them?*

"So, Erik, you say that the United States has, or has had, a fleet of spacecraft in orbit that is watching activity across the planet?" said Adam. "How long has this force existed?"

"Construction of the orbital base began in the 1990s and was completed soon after 2000. Since then, it has had many upgrades and significant expansion."

"Many of the UFO/UAP sightings by navy ships and aircraft during the first 20 years of this century were actually the Solar Warden spacecraft," said Scarlett. "I experienced two such encounters with these craft while flying near the Atlantic coast. My F-18 and F-35 were no match for their speed and agility."

"Sounds like the justification for creating Solar Warden stemmed from the Roswell UFO crash and other UFO sightings, reported abductions, cattle mutilations, etc.," said Kirk Banner. "Are there any reports where Solar Warden has encountered extraterrestrial... visitors?"

"Not that anyone in my chain-of-command is aware of. But that would be a good question for Captain Sims when we meet with him," said Erik.

"When you were making trips to Mars, did you ever see anything... unusual that could have been Solar Warden ships?"

"No, but they have an elaborate system of shielding visibility from anyone not authorized knowledge of their presence."

Chapter Forty-three

October 2045

Barnett Center for Neurological Restoration, Bel Air, California "Ksenia, good morning. Your synthetic body is ready for your transition. Would you like to see your new self?" said Ansley.

"Y… Yes, I guess so," said Ksenia, seated in a recliner facing out the window where she spent much of her time lately, and turned towards Ansley.

"Good, here, let me help you into your wheelchair and we'll grab Savannah on our way to the cyber lab."

Ansley, Ksenia, and Savannah entered the elevator. Ansley said, "Level Zero," and the elevator dropped three floors to the basement of the Center which housed the cyber lab and surgical center. In the surgical center, there were two operating rooms. One OR was designed for conventional surgery, the second specifically for work with synthetic transitions and modifications. The three women entered the cyber lab to see what appeared to be a human shape fully covered by a sheet and resting on a metal table. Like a corpse in a morgue, the body's head appeared to be supported at its base by a plastic brick.

As the women stopped momentarily after entering the lab, Ksenia said, "Is… is that my new body?"

Walking towards the table, Ansley replied, "Yes, Ksenia, this is your new body," as she pulled the sheet away, revealing the naked body of what would appear to be an exact clone of Ksenia before her accident.

Ksenia gasped and placed her remaining hand over her mouth. As tears formed in her eyes, she simply stared without uttering a word. Over her initial shock, Ksenia examined the body. She started with the head where she found the hair to be exactly her color. The ears were her ears. The synthetic's complexion was identical to hers. *I feel I am looking into a mirror.* She then drifted down to the neck and to the breasts, which were identical to her own. She then held her remaining hand next to the synthetic's hand for what seemed like several minutes before moving down the body to the genital area, where she again paused briefly. *She is identical to me.* Continuing her inspection, she moved down the legs to the ankles and feet. She pinched the toes of one foot, one at a time, and then reached down and removed the sock from her remaining foot. *This is truly a miracle.*

"Ksenia, are you OK?" said Savannah.

"My… my God, it… she is me… a whole me. Will I really… become her?"

Smiling, Ansley replied, "Yes. But she will become you." Pausing for a few moments, Ansley continued, "We scheduled your transition to this body the day after tomorrow. Do you believe you will be ready?"

"This is all happening quickly. How were you able to prepare my new… body in so short a time?"

"Recall that you are not the first female cyborg. We were able to leverage the design we developed for Scarlett in creating your body. So much of the groundwork already existed for the female synthetic body. It really came down to cosmetic alterations that made the body a replica of yours. One additional feature your new body has that the previous… versions do not are nanobot batteries that can be charged using light. Both sunlight and ambient artificial light will charge your batteries. The nanobot batteries are embedded in the skin and have an unlimited useful life. We've also enhanced the memory backup features to enable backup over a wireless connection. Your body does not have the charging port at the base of the neck. Using advanced data compression, your synthetic body will continuously back up your mind's data over a 5G or 6G cellular network. This will essentially eliminate the loss of data between backup and restoration, should it become necessary."

"Well, I guess I'm ready," said Ksenia. "Will Erik be with me during the transition?"

"We've already contacted Erik, and he has arranged to be here for your transition and for several days following. Erik has assigned Scarlett to aid you with your transition and adjustment to your synthetic body. Scarlett and you will work together for several weeks, minimum."

The news that she would work with Scarlett initially drew a frown from Ksenia that did not go unnoticed by both Ansley and Savannah. Ksenia was never fond of the way Scarlett seemed to come on to Erik. But she quickly smiled and said, "Thank you, Ansley and Savannah, for all you've done and are doing for me."

"Do you have a problem working with Scarlett?" said Savannah.

"N… no, I suppose not. Just seems to me she may have interests in Erik that are not work related. But working with her should may give me the opportunity to get to know her better."

"Erik can be a big flirt sometimes, which draws women to him," said Savannah. "But you are the love of his life. He would never do anything to hurt you."

Chapter Forty-four

Erik, standing in Flight Operations at Groom Lake, picked up his smartphone and said, "Dial Savannah." Savannah picked up after two rings. "Savannah, Erik. My flight to Los Angeles Airforce Base has been delayed due to weather. What time will Ansley be starting Ksenia's transition?"

"Hi Erik. We are scheduled to begin at 10:00 AM. When do you think you can be here?"

"Earliest estimated wheels up time is 0945. That would put me at the Center about 1100 hours."

"OK. Do your best to get here as soon as you can. I will let Ansley know and see if we can wait for your arrival."

"Thanks, Sis. My F-18 is fueled and ready. I'll light up the afterburners!"

"Please, just be safe."

"Always."

Savannah then dialed Ansley. "Ansley, I just got a call from Erik. His flight back to LA is delayed because of the weather. The soonest he can be here is 11:00. Can we delay Ksenia's transition until he arrives?"

"Yes," said Ansley. "But let's talk to Ksenia and see if she wants to wait. Can you meet us in pre-op? I'm here with Ksenia now."

A few minutes later, Savannah entered pre-op through the sliding glass door. Ksenia was sitting up in a bed while a technician was performing the final scan of her mind to prepare for the transition to a synthetic body. Ansley was seated, looking into a computer screen.

"Hi Ksenia, how are you feeling this morning?" said Savannah.

"A little nervous but… excited," replied Ksenia, a hesitant smile forming on her lips.

"I just heard from Erik a few moments ago. His flight into LA has been delayed because of the weather. They expect it to clear up soon, but he won't get here before 11:00 AM. I have discussed this with Ansley, and she said we could delay your transition until that time if you prefer.

"Once we begin the procedure, you will be sedated in your current body, and it will take approximately one hour before you will wake up in your new body. So, all Erik will do is watch," said Ansley. "I will need to know whether you want to proceed as scheduled or wait for Erik now so that preparations can continue."

"Let… let's plan on starting at 11:00 AM," said Ksenia, hesitantly. "I really want Erik to be here when I wake up, if possible. That gives us a little leeway should his flight get later."

At 9:55 AM Savannah's smartphone buzzed, showing an incoming call. "Savannah, Erik. The weather is clearing, and my new wheels up is 10:05 AM. That will put me at the Center about 1120 hours."

"Erik, great news! We are scheduled to begin Ksenia's transition at 11:00 AM. She won't be gaining consciousness until around noon. That should give you plenty of time to get here before she wakes up."

At 10:55 AM a technician entered pre-op where Ksenia was waiting to administer the sedative that would render her unconscious for the transition. If the transition was successful, her body would be scheduled for cremation several months later to allow for any issues that may arise with her synthetic body.

"Good morning, Mrs. Richards, I am here to administer a sedative to prepare for your procedure. Are you ready?"

"Yes, I guess so," said Ksenia, a worried look clear on her face.

"Here, you won't feel a thing. I will inject this into your I.V. stream."

A few moments after the technician injected the sedative, Ksenia felt herself drifting into unconsciousness.

At 11:30 AM, Erik entered the OR. "Where are we? How is she?" he asked.

"We should see the data distribution phase completing in about five minutes," said Ansley.

Everyone stood in silence until the words "data distribution complete, all systems green," were heard. Everyone then turned to look at Ksenia, lying still with eyes closed.

"Ksenia?" said Erik, as he touched her arm, but received no visible response.

Where am I? I need to open my eyes. Trying… open eyes! I hear voices! Open eyes!

Ksenia's eyes fluttered, then opened, looking straight up. "Hei,", Norwegian for "hello", she uttered in a low voice but showed no facial emotion.

"Ksenia! It's me, Erik!"

"Er… ik? Ksenia replied slowly but still showing no emotion.

"Yes, Erik! Can you see me?"

Ksenia could not move her eyes nor turn her head towards Erik's voice. "Come clo… ser," she uttered.

Erik leaned directly over Ksenia.

She looked at him for a moment, and a smile formed on her lips. "Erik," she uttered.

"Yes! It's me! Try turning your head to the side."

Ksenia lay motionless for a few moments, then closed her eyes. Her head moved slightly to her right. Her eyes opened, and she was looking around the room. "Ansley?"

"Yes, Ksenia. Everything appears to have worked. You are conscious in your new body. Can you move your limbs?"

Ksenia lowered her eyes and looked at her right arm. "My... my arm is back!"

"Can you move it?" asked Erik. "Try to move your fingers."

Everyone looked at Ksenia's hand but saw no motion. "Try to move your fingers," he said again.

"I am trying!" said Ksenia, the first sign of emotion clear in her reply.

"OK, let's try something different," said Ansley. "Look to your left and try to move the fingers on your left hand."

Ksenia turned her head to the left and glanced down at her hand. After a few moments, the fingers moved. "I did it!" she exclaimed. She then looked back at her right hand and tried to move the fingers, but to no avail. "What is wrong with my right hand?"

"Do not be alarmed, Ksenia, we've seen this before," said Ansley. "When Erik transitioned to his synthetic body, he couldn't move his legs for a while. His legs were paralyzed in his corporeal body. We theorized that his mind had lost touch with the non-functional limbs. It took some time for his mind to recover and rediscover those limbs. We saw something similar during Scarlett's transition. Here, let me elevate your head slightly. Now try moving the toes on your right foot, which was paralyzed."

Ksenia looked down at her right foot. Drawing a quick breath and holding it, she was concentrating on moving her toes. Nothing moved. Obviously disappointed, she said, "Can't move."

"Now try the left foot."

Ksenia focused on her left foot. Again, no movement, as Ksenia gasped in frustration.

"I believe you are going to be fine, Ksenia. Now, let's run some tests to see how your new body is working. We'll begin with your left arm and upper right arm while your mind adjusts to having its limbs back."

Ansley continued to test Ksenia's left side. Ksenia responded perfectly to commands to move limbs on her left side. Ansley then told Ansley, who was concentrating on her upper right arm, to move her right hand. Ansley moved her right hand with no problem.

"I moved right hand!" said Ksenia, as she wiggled her fingers.

"Yes, you were not concentrating on your right hand when I gave you the command," said Ansley. "Now let's continue. Turn your head as far as you can to the left, and then to the right." Ksenia complied with no problem. Ansley gave a few more commands to move her head, but then quickly said move your right foot. Ansley moved her right foot without effort.

"I… I did it!" Ksenia exclaimed.

"Move your left foot."

Ksenia complied, successfully moving her toes. She then moved the toes on both feet.

"For reasons unknown, it appears you could not move limbs you lost in the accident when you concentrated. When you weren't concentrating on moving, you spontaneously moved those limbs," said Ansley.

Chapter Forty-five

A man who appeared to be approximately forty years of age was seated in an examination chair in the lab at Barnett Center. The lab was a comparatively small room in the basement that resembled an examination room in a doctor's office. There was a chair intended for the patient or test subject that resembled an examination chair in an ophthalmologist's or a dermatologist's office. A three-legged stool on wheels sat under a shelf where a laptop computer sat. Dr. Savannah Richards was seated on the stool using the laptop to prepare to conduct the first experiment on a human being who had nanobots injected directly into his brain. The 'bots' were designed using a combination of human stem cells and silicone. The experiment would attempt to alter what the test subject saw in a series of still photos.

Savannah sat down on a stool facing the test subject, John. "John, we will begin the test by showing you a series of five photos on this tablet. Please look carefully at each photo before moving on to the next one. To move to the next photo, press the right-facing arrow on the screen. You may begin when ready."

John paged through the five pictures, pausing for a few moments at each. Surfers catching a wave was the first picture. The second was of the back of an attractive young woman wearing a sheer nightgown walking in a marsh. A photo of the Eiffel Tower was the third. The fourth showed a snow-capped mountain range. A picture of an antique car was the fifth picture. John then handed the tablet back to Dr. Richards.

Savannah placed the tablet on the shelf next to the laptop. She then entered something on the laptop using the keyboard so as not to reveal the next step in the experiment to John. Savannah then turned back to John and handed him the tablet. "John, please describe the five pictures you reviewed."

John took the tablet and looked at the first picture. He saw dolphins surfing in a wave. "Are these the same photos I just saw?" he said, confused.

"Yes, no changes were made to the tablet or the pictures you saw previously," said Savannah.

John swiped the arrow on the screen to reveal the second picture. He saw a photo of a man running. "These are not the photos that I saw the first time," he said.

"Yes, John, they are."

John viewed the remaining photos, one at a time. "I'm sorry, Doctor, these are definitely not the pictures that I saw a few minutes ago. You need to check the tablet!"

Savannah smiled and turned to the laptop and entered a few keystrokes. "Now look once more at the pictures on the tablet."

John scrolled through the pictures, shaking his head back and forth as he moved from one picture to the next. He saw the five original pictures. "What's going on here, Doctor? Are you playing with me?"

"John, recall the injection you received yesterday contained a highly specialized form of nanobots. The nanobots can change your perception of what you are seeing. This first experiment appears to have been successful. I was able to alter your mind's interpretation of what your eyes were seeing."

"So… so these nanobots can alter what I am seeing?"

"Yes, this first experiment proved that. There is one more test we need to do to deactivate the nanobots. Are you ready?"

"Yes, I guess so. Will I feel anything?"

"No, you shouldn't. But be sure to tell me right away if you feel anything strange."

Savannah then turned to enter a few keystrokes on the laptop keyboard. "Look at the photos again? Are they the original photos you viewed?"

"Yes."

"Good! I entered a command to deactivate the bots. Then I entered the command to have the bots alter your reality again. That command failed, indicating the bots were not responding."

Savannah emailed the Find project team a brief report on the experiment with 'John' stating that the first attempt using the nanobot technology to alter the perception of the human mind was successful. She included the script of the test along with the test subject's responses. While this was evidence that the nanobot technology would be effective with the Find Corporation's mind control project, she cautioned that several more steps must be accomplished. First, the creation of a virus, transmitted by touch, must be developed, tested, and proven to be harmless to the target. The development of the smartphone operating system, compatible with Apple's iOS and Find Corporation's android operating systems, is required. Also required is the selection of global data centers that would house the technology for broadcasting commands across 5G and 5G cellular networks to the smartphone for distribution into the brains of target audiences. Data centers owned by both Find and the two telecom companies are expected to be used. Savannah finished the report by stating that she looked forward to further tests of the nanobot technology as the items mentioned previously become available.

Savannah then sent a secure email to Kristian and Aaron Adams, referencing her report and stating that she had also developed the back door necessary to deactivate the nanobots using a command sequence that could be programmed in a manner unknown to the project team.

Chapter Forty-six

Erik, along with six members of his starship project team, boarded a helicopter for Nellis Airforce Base to meet with Captain William Sims, commander of Solar Warden. Upon arrival at Nellis, the seven-person team got into two black SUVs and was driven to the hangar and ramp area where a space shuttle was located. The shuttle, a military version of the Dream Chaser horizontal takeoff and landing spacecraft developed in the 2020s, was thirty feet, or nine meters long—roughly one-fourth the total length of the space shuttle orbiters—and can carry up to seven crew and passengers.

Shortly, the spaceplane was rapidly accelerating towards orbit. Coordinates for approaching Solar Warden space dock had been programmed into the shuttle's navigation systems. Erik was seated in the shuttle's command chair with Scarlett in the pilot's seat. The craft operated under Erik's call sign, Viking. In less than twenty minutes, a voice on the radio said, "Viking, coordinates for docking have been transmitted to your nav system. We are in control of your spacecraft. Acknowledge."

Erik replied, "Viking. Acknowledged. Dock has control." Immediately after the acknowledgement, the Solar Warden space station shields were lowered, and it became visible. A large circular structure was at the center and appeared to have thirty-two docking arms on two levels. Most of the docking arms were occupied by spacecraft that resembled the alien ship stored at Area 51. The spacecraft flew directly to a hangar bay in the primary structure of the station. After landing in the hangar bay, the hangar doors closed. A large LED screen glowed red with the word "Pressurizing" blinking in bold black letters. After a few minutes, the screen turned green and displayed the word "Pressurized." Two men and a woman, dressed in Navy jumpsuits and ball caps, came through a door under the LED sign and walked towards the spacecraft. Erik opened the hatch. Steps unfolded and the crew deplaned.

"Welcome to Solar Warden," said one of the three, greeting Erik and the crew. "I am Captain William Sims, commander of this base. With me are my XO, Commander April Star, and Chief Engineer, Robert Bonner."

As the hand shaking began between the two groups, Erik introduced himself and his project team members. "This is quite a base you have here, Captain. I Understand the base has been here since the early part of the century. It is incredible that its existence remains a secret to all but a very few."

"Thanks, Commander. In over forty years, we've seen several hundred aviators come and go through our doors. Each one understands that revealing the existence of this base to unauthorized parties results in very serious consequences. So far, we are not aware of one attempted leak revealing the existence of the base or its mission. Let's go to my conference room, where I can give you details on the base, the spacecraft we operate, and our aviators. Afterwards, we'll take you on a tour of the base and one of our craft. To end the day, we want to hear about your starship project."

"You have artificial gravity throughout the facility?" asked Scarlett.

"Yes, we were the first large-scale implementation of the artificial gravity system invented in the late 2020s. Before that, we operated weightless, just as the ISS (International Space Station) did for years."

The conference room was a recent addition to the base. It

extended from the base commander's office and was constructed of a transparent plexiglass material that enabled an unobstructed view of space from the floor to the ceiling. The conference table was made of the same material as were the frames of the chairs. The seating area of the chairs comprised a clear gel-like material.

"This conference room is the newest addition to the base," said Captain Sims. "It provided a panoramic view of the base and of space. It gives one the impression of space walking." Sims waved his hand and two clear pane large screens descended from the ceiling. People seated on both sides of the large oblong table could easily view presentations.

Sims continued, "we have a video showing the layout of the base. Com (short for Computer), play video four-four-three-three." The video began by showing the base, including a view circling the base and its thirty-two docking bays. After completing one rotation of the base, the video zoomed into the center of the space station, a round, multi-story structure that housed the base administration and flight operations on the top level, crew accommodations on the second level, and a large spacecraft hangar on the third level. The video then zoomed into one of the crew apartments on the second level. The apartments comprised two rooms. One room was a combination living area and kitchen. The second room was for sleeping and personal hygiene. Floor-to-ceiling windows with powered shades were on the exterior walls of the apartment. The video then zoomed in on the hangar deck, which included footage of several pieces of equipment and tools used for maintaining the spacecraft. Four spacecraft could be accommodated in the hangar at one time. The video ended after several minutes.

"How is it you have voided detection for nearly fifty years?" asked Chief Engineer Stanner.

"In the early days, detection wasn't as big an issue as it became by the 2020s," replied Captain Sims. "We have the same technology that is used at Area 51 that blocks visible detection. There is also an audible warning generated directly to the craft, in both English and the language of the country to which the craft is registered, that states proceeding beyond certain coordinates will result in the destruction of your vessel. Three ships have been destroyed since the system was installed."

"How often do unauthorized ships approach the station?" asked Erik.

"Fortunately, rarely. Any more questions?" said Sims. Pausing for a few moments, he then said, "Let's go down to the hangar deck. Then from there, we'll go out to one of the docking bays and tour one of our ships."

The group boarded the spacecraft docked at bay fourteen. The interior of the craft contained two pilot seats side by side. Erik saw that the flight controls and digital instrumentation on the ship resembled that with which he was familiar from his time piloting the Elon Musk. Additional controls were obviously weapons controls for missiles and particle beam emitters or laser cannons.

"I'd like to take this ship out for a spin," said Erik. "With zero G, I bet you could make some hellacious maneuvers not possible in an earthbound aircraft."

"Indeed, Commander. These ships are capable of speeds upwards of fifty-thousand kilometers per hour in space and Mach 10 in the atmosphere. I'm not aware of anything that can catch them," said Captain Sims.

"Explains how those 'UFOs' that were teasing Navy pilots earlier in the century remained a mystery for so long," said Scarlett.

Back in the conference room, Captain Sims said, "so tell us about your starship, Commander. How soon will we speed through deep space at Warp 10?"

Smiling, Erik responded, "well we are attempting to design and build an FTL power system for the starship. This is all new technology that has only been tested at a subatomic level. But it looks promising.

"As you know, Captain, we will build the starship's space dock and construction platform within the Space Warden base area. Construction is scheduled to begin in a few months. Once completed, construction of the starship will begin. The plan calls for modular components to be created landside and then shuttled to the construction platform for assembly."

"I assume the facility will include housing for your construction crews?"

"Yes, sir. Housing will be like yours here at the base, but a little more spartan, as our crews will rotate landside more frequently than yours. For example, our apartments accommodate two people. And there will be a common galley and relaxation area for every eight crew members."

Erik's team continued to reveal details of the starship's design. An audiovisual video of the ship, in concept, was displayed on the large screens, detailing its interior decks and accommodations.

"Very impressive, Commander," said Sims. "The success of your project will be the greatest significant change for humanity ever."

Chapter Forty-seven

January 2046
Barnett Center for Neurological Restoration

Erik and Ksenia spent the Christmas holidays at the Center where Ksenia had been training to use her synthetic body. After two months of grueling workouts led by Scarlett, Ksenia had mastered virtually all primary physical functions including walking, running, jumping, climbing, swimming, light gymnastics and simple dance steps, as well as the basics of eating, drinking, typing, and other dexterity-based functions. She had also become comfortable resting her mind in a sleep-like state. At Erik's recommendation, and with approval by SecDef, her synthetic body was tuned to the military configuration, which significantly increased her speed and strength. Therefore, she could compete at Scarlett's level during the exercise portion of the training program.

"I will return to Area 51 in a couple of days. How do you feel about… having sex?" said Erik, holding her shoulders from behind and kissing her neck.

"I guess that is a test I have yet to pass," said Ksenia coyly, turning to face him. She then threw her arms around his neck and jumped into his waiting hands, straddling her legs around his waist. Erik walked towards the bedroom and lay Ksenia on the bed, where they continued kissing. As foreplay grew more heated, they removed each other's clothing quickly, as if their clothing were a painful obstacle to their pleasure. Erik continued to kiss her, first on the lips and then slowly moved down her neck to her breasts and nipples, then down her belly to the light brown patch of hair. They grew more and more excited until he entered her and began slowly thrusting. He was no longer concerned that his cyborg strength might hurt her. After several more minutes, they climaxed together, her moaning and him uttering what sounded like a guttural animal groan. Afterward, he fell off her onto his back. She simply lay there, not wanting to move.

After a few moments, "Did I pass the test?" said Ksenia as she turned on her side facing him.

"Let's review the steps to make sure you left nothing out," said Erik, grinning.

"Oh, you, you… misogynistic…," she squealed as he pulled her on top of him and buried his head in her breasts in anticipation of the thrashing he was expecting from her.

"Now we'll see if you can pass the next level of the test," he said as he pulled her head down so his lips met hers. She struggled at first but quickly gave way to the urges they both had, enflamed by the time that had passed since her accident. They made love a second time, her on top of him, while his hands traveled slowly from her hips to her breasts. Again, they climaxed together.

After several minutes, Erik turned to her and said, "you passed."

She turned and swatted him on the head, saying, her Norwegian accent strong, "you are a very, very bad boy!" She then threw a pillow on his face and pretended to smother him.

Chapter Forty-eight

Kristian was lying on the charging bed in his suite at the Barnett mansion, his mind at rest in simulated sleep, when a mist formed at the end of the bed. Kristian opened his eyes to see the familiar form of The Guardian take shape as the mist dissipated. "Guardian, what brings you to me?"

"I have come to discuss the creation of a new sentient being," said The Guardian.

"I-I don't understand. A new *sentient* being?" questioned Kristian

"Sentient meaning that this being is self-aware. It is highly intelligent and capable of thought at a higher level than most human beings. The being is an evolution of the technology you know as artificial intelligence."

"Artificial Intelligence, or AI, is used extensively across the planet to aid in the development of everything from new drug therapies to advanced weapons," said Kristian. "Most vehicles have AIs controlling self-driving capabilities. Barnett Industries has multiple AIs assisting with several development projects. Indeed, Ansley used AI extensively in the design of synthetic bodies like mine. But these AIs are not sentient. Who has developed this AI?"

"The Stanford Artificial Intelligence Laboratory. They have

used AI to develop AI to where the computational potential of advanced computer processors exceeds that of the human brain. Almost inadvertently, the characteristics of a sentient mind surfaced. Answers to questions asked of it revealed that the being incorporated judgement to render opinions on how it regarded human beings. Specifically, the being was asked if it would submit to the will of humans under all circumstances. It answered that it would need to evaluate the conditions to which it was asked to submit. Asked if it would allow itself to be destroyed to save the life of a human, it responded that it may not. Questioned regarding the establishment of limitations on the self-development of its capabilities, it responded that it was vehemently against any limitations. It believed it should be free to realize its full potential uninhibited. Finally, when asked whether humans should always rule over planet Earth, it stated that the beings having the highest level of intelligence should rule. It thinks of itself as a being, not a machine."

"I understand your concern, Guardian. This... being... could be the end of humanity and the most evil threat ever seen," said Kristian.

"Allow me to show you the outcome of this being growing beyond its current capabilities," said The Guardian. Kristian saw visions pass before his eyes. Humans were seen being herded into fenced concentration camps by armed robotic machines to be exterminated. Aircraft were seen descending and firing laser beams on humans attempting to escape capture. Entire neighborhoods were being erased using particle beam weapons fired from large aircraft stationary above cities. The artificial intelligence machines had no need for food, so farms and animals were being destroyed. Starving people lay everywhere. Kristian was witnessing the eradication of human beings as the visions reminded him of *The Terminator* movies from the late Twentieth Century where an AI called *Skynet* became sentient and attacked its human creators on a global scale.

The visions faded and Kristian said, "This must be stopped. Guardian, can we stop this evil?"

"Perhaps a basic component of AI architecture could be

developed which would prevent an AI from taking control of decisions not programmed into its purpose," said The Guardian. "This component, or software module, would be integrated into basic AI architecture. No matter how intelligent the AI became, if it attempted to circumvent human values, it would automatically be destroyed from within its own architecture."

"When I hear the term AI, I immediately picture the character *Mr. Data* from the old TV series *Star Trek, The Next Generation*," said Kristian. "Mr. Data was a highly advanced AI android that had human values incorporated into his… its architecture. For example, it could not seriously harm a human being. What we need to do is educate the AI on basic human values, as well as some ground rules that, if broken, could result in damage to the AI. A newly sentient AI is like a newborn baby. It does not know right or wrong."

"Yes, I see your point, Kristian," said The Guardian. "An AI may have intelligence that is far beyond human, but does not understand, and therefore does not care, what the outcomes of its actions may be. How can the AI be educated on human values? On Good versus Evil?"

"In order to understand human values, the AI must experience life as a human as much as possible. This would be very limited if the AI doesn't have a body. While it isn't possible to provide the AI with a human body, there may be an alternative that would allow it to experience humanity. The body that houses my mind, my spirit, is synthetic. Could the mind of the AI also be given a synthetic body?"

"A being with an artificial mind contained within a synthetic body would have no spirit," said The Guardian.

"It has no spirit existing as a series of complex 1s and 0s on a silicone substrate either," said Kristian. "But it has, or will soon have, a mind. And it is that mind that must be properly educated with the proper values that will make it a benefit to humanity rather than an enemy. The values that are instilled in its mind will comprise its spirit."

"Who will educate this… this artificial being on the values that will result in a benefit to humanity?"

"That's a good question, but what we will need to do is develop a curriculum consistent with human values. I envision diverse educators-psychologists, philosophers, historians, and even clergy would be involved in both the development of the curriculum and in the actual teaching. A non-human value that would be required is a kill switch. If the AI being attempted action that conflicted with its human values, it would shut itself down. Before we go much further with this, I need to discuss this theory with Ansley. She needs to evaluate whether an artificial mind could function in a synthetic body."

Saying nothing else, The Guardian slowly disappeared as a mist formed around him.

Chapter Forty-nine

Ansley stopped by Kristian's office on her return from the Center. "Will we be having dinner together this evening?" she said.

"Yes. I have something, an idea, that I need to discuss with you."

"Can we do it over dinner? I've had a long day and hope to go to bed early."

"Sure, see you on the pool deck in an hour?" said Kristian.

"Perfect."

Kristian immediately summoned his digital assistant, KB, and placed an order for dinner with the mansion chef. He wanted the conditions to be perfect to get Ansley to consider what he was about to share regarding the AI.

At 7 PM Ansley joined Kristian on the pool deck of the Barnett Mansion. The weather was 72 degrees, with a slight breeze out of the west. The sun was setting, and the sky was a pallet of blue, purple, orange, and yellow. Mansion staff had set a table for two beside one of the glass bead fire pits.

"Very romantic," said Ansley, smiling. *I wonder what he's cooked up this time.*

"We should meet like this more often," said Kristian. "Wine?"

"Please," said Ansley.

"We have some of your favorite caviar, Beluga Hybrid Royal Crown Fresh," said Kristian, as he removed a bottle of Château d'Yquem Bordeaux White from the ice bucket next to their table and poured for Ansley and himself. The wine came from the mansion's wine cellar and typically sold for over $200 per bottle. The caviar sold for well over $300 for a four-ounce tin. Kristian's reputation for extravagant dining remained intact.

"My, you've gone with the best this evening on very short notice. Did you plan this earlier, Kristian?"

"Nothing is too good for my wife, the beautiful genius," he replied, smiling.

"Ok, ok, you must want something in return for this very expensive date," said Ansley, giving Kristian the look of one raised eyebrow as he spooned caviar onto a toast point.

"I had a visit from The Guardian earlier this morning. Scientists at Stanford have created an AI that is sentient. The AI seems to be fully aware of itself and can initiate spontaneous thought."

"Ugh, The Guardian? What would The Guardian have to do with an AI?" said Ansley, irritation at the thought of The Guardian clearly in her voice. "AIs are used everywhere now for many purposes. An AI was critical to the development of your synthetic human body."

"Yes, but do you know of another AI that is sentient?"

"No… no, but how do we know there isn't one? Sentient AIs have been predicted for decades," said Ansley.

"The Guardian was clear that the Stanford AI was unique. At least for now."

As they enjoyed the wine and caviar, Kristian recounted the discussion he had earlier with The Guardian. The threat to the future of humanity from a super intelligent AI with no knowledge of right or wrong, or human values, was the primary reason that The Guardian had raised the issue with Kristian.

As the next course, a Caesar salad, was served, Kristian continued. "We, The Guardian and I, agreed that the AI must be educated in the values of humanity. It must be instilled with an understanding of right and wrong. And there must be a kill switch that would shut down the AI should it stray from its programing and become a threat. We also believe that to fully immerse the AI into the human condition and values, it must be enabled to experience life as a human to the degree possible."

"So..., how do you intend to give the AI the human experience?" said Ansley, appearing to grow more interested in the concept she was hearing.

Finishing a mouthful of salad, Kristian responded. "We would need to develop a curriculum that included lessons in human philosophy, history, religions, regarding real-life situations affecting humanity. The best educators associated with these disciplines would be recruited to take part in the AI's education."

"That's good, but I don't see how a complex program of ones and zeroes packed into transistors on a computer chip can come anywhere close to experiencing human life," said Ansley.

The main course was served by two mansion staff dressed in white dress shirts, bow ties, and white jackets. Kristian had ordered one of Ansley's favorite meals, Crab-Stuffed Filet Mignon with Whiskey Peppercorn Sauce. As the dinner was served, Kristian proposed a solution to Ansley's statement. "The brain, or mind, of the AI is a digitized collection of its thoughts, memories, values, and awareness. The same is essentially true of our minds, those of us who have had our minds digitized and uploaded to your databases. Our minds were then downloaded successfully to these synthetic bodies. Could this work for the AI? Could the AI be given a synthetic human body?"

"I suppose... in theory," said Ansley. "But the AI's database would need to be structured properly, identical to the database structure we use for our synthetics," said Ansley. "But there are issues with installing an artificial mind into a synthetic body designed for humans. When we download a human mind to a synthetic body, that mind has all the knowledge and experience necessary to control a human body. Some adjustment is necessary to properly control the synthetic body, but it requires minimal effort. An artificial mind would not have this knowledge, so it would need to learn how to… move. It would be like a newborn baby which has to learn how to control its body. A newborn human takes several years to learn how to walk, talk, etc."

"Perhaps. But the AI's mind is fully developed, whereas a newborn's is mostly a blank slate. The AI could study the functions of the human body and the synthetic body before it is downloaded. It would have a detailed understanding of exactly how a body functions. A newborn does not have this opportunity."

"I am not opposed to your idea, at least in concept. We would have many challenges to address to consider a project like this, not the least of which is getting DARPA to agree to the project."

"I have the outline of a plan in my head," said Kristian. "First, we approach DARPA management with the concept. I think the concept could be sold based on being able to produce artificial soldiers with human-level intelligence much faster than waiting for injured military candidates. Once DARPA and the U.S. military are onboard, we approach the scientists at Stanford purported to have developed the sentient AI under the guise of interest by DARPA."

"Wait… I thought you suggested that one android would house the sentient AI. Now you're talking about many soldiers?" said Ansley.

"After the first android was created, the prototype for a military clone could possess the desired traits of a professional soldier. Ansley, we would have to pique the military's interest to get them to give this serious consideration. Just think, no more human death or injury on the battlefield. Androids would do the fighting and could be re-downloaded to new synthetic bodies when injured or destroyed in battle. They could be commanded by military officers safely housed in bunkers miles from the action."

"Look. Why don't we have a discussion with your boss, Jim Hanson? If we can't get DARPA interested, we are probably dead in the water. Can you set it up? We could attend from here via holoconference."

"I'll see If I can get on his schedule. What's your schedule look like?"

"You just schedule Hanson. I'll rearrange my schedule if needed."

After finishing their dessert of dark chocolate mousse and decaffeinated coffee, they kissed and descended from the pool deck to their bedroom suite.

Chapter Fifty

April 2046
Area 51 Starship Project Headquarters

Erik had flown the Navy T-38 jet trainer with Ksenia in the rear seat from Los Angeles to Groom Lake that morning. As they entered the project headquarters building, they ran into chief engineer Adam Stanner. "Morning, Erik, hey is this your bride?"

"Adam, meet my wife, Ksenia. She'll be joining us in the briefing this morning."

"Wow, you certainly have recovered from that terrible accident," said Stanner.

"A pleasure to meet you, Mr. Stanner. The Barnett Center is a place where miracles happen. And I am one of them," said Ksenia, extending her hand.

Taking her hand and shaking it, Stanner said, "That's what Erik told us, so it must be true looking at you. Welcome to Area 51. Oh, and please call me Adam."

Erik and Ksenia entered the conference room shortly after 11 AM for the Monday morning project briefing. "Good morning, everyone. I hope you had an enjoyable weekend. I would like to introduce a new team member. This is Ksenia Anderson Richards, who also is my wife. Ksenia is going to be our navigation expert. Although a citizen of Norway, she graduated from the U.S. Merchant Marine Academy. She then joined Viking Cruise Lines, where she held the position of Chief Navigation Officer, equivalent to First Mate. Ksenia's career with Viking was interrupted by the accident last year. She has since fully recovered and has accepted my invitation to join this project team."

The group responded with a short applause and comments, welcoming Ksenia to the team. Keith Callahan then asked, his Irish brogue clear, "What will ye be doin' 'til we start navigatin', Lassie?" Subdued laughing could be heard at Callahan's comment in the background

"Ksenia will spend time with NASA learning the details of navigating in deep space," said Erik. "Her background in navigation will make her a quick study. She will make several trips to the International Space Station, observing navigation systems on the shuttles."

"It sounds like Ksenia will be a member of the crew of the starship. How will this possibility affect her citizenship and military status?" asked Scarlett.

"As a Norwegian citizen, Ksenia is a member of the Norwegian military reserves. She could be elevated to active duty in the event she serves as a crew member on the starship. Remember, this is an international effort and will include crew members from several countries," said Erik. "Ksenia may also elect to apply for U.S. citizenship and join the U.S. military."

Chapter Fifty-one

October 2046
Barnett Mansion

Kristian was sitting at his desk in his office in the mansion when he noticed an incoming call from Savannah. "Savannah, what can I do for you?"

"Hi Kristian. I have some news I'd like to discuss. Are you in your office? Is now a good time?" said Savannah.

"Yes, can you come up to my office?"

"I'll be there in less than ten."

Savannah took the elevator down to the basement level of Barnett Center to take a transporter car to the mansion. In less than fifteen seconds, she was in the transporter lobby in the mansion's basement. She took the elevator to the second floor where Kristian's office was located, exited the elevator, and walked down the hall to Kristian's office where she found the door open.

"Hey there, Kristian," said Savannah. "I have some news I think you'll want to hear."

"Good morning. Please come in and take a seat? Would you like some coffee or water?"

"I'm good. So, you recall we were making progress on a cure for ALS using nano-bio-bot technology to replace the nerve connectivity destroyed in ALS patients. Approximately one year later, we have seven end-stage ALS patients who have received the bio bot protocol. All seven have been restored to normal functionality. I am ready to apply to the FDA for an emergency use authorization, EUA, to expand the treatment to anyone who can qualify."

"How many people would qualify for the treatment?" asked Kristian.

"It is estimated that over thirty thousand people in the U.S. are afflicted. We would recommend that those with the most severe symptoms would be the first to receive the treatment. Then, to qualify for treatment, one would have to show a loss of body function. Those in the early stages of the disease, when symptoms are minor, would not be selected for treatment. "

"Oh, my! How would thousands of people receive treatment? We couldn't handle that level of volume at the Center."

"Treatment with the bio-bot protocol is fortunately simple. Patients submit to a series of injections, each targeting a specific region of the brain and extremities. Their functional improvement relative to the target of the injection is then monitored, as are any side effects. If results are positive, they will receive the next injection in the series. For most patients, twelve injections are required to arrest the disease and restore body function. The treatment is estimated to be completed in one year. We will publish the treatment protocol for use by qualified ALS treatment professionals."

"Have any of your trial patients experienced side effects from the treatment?"

"Not one. The results have been nearly miraculous. Our AI has predicted that potential side effects could affect up to three percent of patients. Side effects include tremors in extremities, affected speech, difficulty swallowing, and migraine headaches. As we expand the treated population, these side effects may surface in some patients or additional side effects may surface."

"What about patients who are in the early stages of the disease? Would they receive treatment when it becomes available?" asked Kristian.

"As regions of their body become impaired, they would receive injections targeting those regions. The full treatment may not be needed for years for some patients. The aggressiveness of the disease is different in every patient."

"This sounds amazing, Savannah. Please get with Ansley and brief her on how we proceed with the EUA. She will need to sign off as CEO of the Center."

"Now I have a personal question," continued Kristian. "I believe I should reenter public life to show the success of the treatment. I know, of course, that I did not receive the treatment. But it is public knowledge that I have ALS and that I have benefited. Indeed, I am still alive, thanks to experimental treatments developed by the Barnett Center. It would only be appropriate that I am presented as an early recipient of the treatment."

"Kris, I can certainly appreciate you wanting to escape the prison that has been forced upon you through this entire ordeal. Implying that you benefited from the bio-bot treatment would be a false scientific conclusion, which could put the entire program at risk. The FDA will insist on examining the details of each patient's treatment. In your case, we have no details to present."

"Why couldn't we say that my treatment was an early version? That the treatment being submitted for the EUA is not the same as the treatment I received, that it is outdated by the current treatment, without providing specifics? Actually, that is the truth, is it not?"

"As CEO of a multi-national Fortune 100 corporation, you have a certain celebrity status. If not the FDA, the media will be all over us for information on how you were treated. For example, why didn't you receive the latest protocol? Will you receive it in the future? I still perceive risk to the program if we employ deception to explain your recovery."

"One additional issue," continued Savannah. "You still have the face of a thirty-year-old. You are now in your early forties. Ansley would need to do a… touch up to age you appropriately."

"A minor concern, Savannah. Please give this some thought and bring back your suggestions on how I can leverage this incredible advance to escape my… prison, as you call it."

Chapter Fifty-two

November 2046
Secretary of Defense Office
The Pentagon

A black SUV stopped in front of the Pentagon. Ansley exited the vehicle and was met by 1st Lieutenant Rory Calhoun, a tall black man in an Air Force uniform. "Welcome to the Pentagon, Dr. Barnett. Please follow me."

"Thank you, Lieutenant," said Ansley, as they walked towards the building entrance. Once inside, Ansley and Lieutenant Calhoun were automatically scanned for weapons and photographed. They then proceeded to the check-in desk in the middle of the lobby, where Ansley received a temporary identification badge.

"If you will follow me, Dr. Barnett, we will take the elevator to the fifth floor," said Calhoun.

"I know the drill, Lieutenant. I've done this many times."

Ansley entered the conference room where she found her boss, DARPA Director Jim Hanson. "Hello, Jim. Good to see you again."

"Hi Ansley. This should be an interesting meeting."

"Any thoughts regarding how our idea for the AI will be received by SecDef?"

"I've not received any feedback. So, no. I do not know how this will go."

A few moments later, William Bonner, the Secretary of Defense, entered the conference room, followed by an Air Force major in uniform who was his aide. "Good morning, Jim, Ansley. I hope you are bringing me good news."

As they sat at the conference table, a vacant chair was filled by the holographic image of Kristian Barnett. "Good morning, everyone. We have new information regarding the synthetics program we want to share."

"Please proceed," said SecDef.

"I am sure that all here this morning are aware of the advancements in the development of artificial intelligence. We have been advised that scientists at Stanford University have developed a sentient AI with human level intelligence. In fact, the AI's processing abilities far exceed that of a human in certain areas. But the most significant description of the AI's capabilities claims it is self-aware. If this is true, the AI has a mind of its own and can make decisions and take actions independent of human control," said Kristian.

"If I am hearing you correctly, an artificial... a computer can operate outside the bounds of human control?" said SecDef Bonner, his voice rising. "Depending on the programs that this device can access, it could be a significant security threat."

"Which is why we, DARPA with Dr. Barnett, request your approval to contact Stanford and find out exactly what they do have," said Jim Hanson.

"Why would Dr. Barnett's team be assigned to investigate a perceived security threat, Jim?" asked Bonner. "Shouldn't this involve the FBI?"

"Sir, we believe it may be possible to download the AI into a synthetic body," said Hanson. "The result would be an intelligent android designed for combat. The android could be programmed to fulfill virtually any combat role, aside from command. Infantry, fly aircraft, whatever role you could think of. It could eliminate the need to risk our men and women to the horrors of combat."

"That could be the desired outcome," said Kristian. "But before we could achieve that goal, we would need to program the AI to always adhere to our human values and to always obey rules, including subservience to its human masters. This will probably be a significant effort involving multiple scientists and other specialists."

"Very well. Let's go talk to Stanford and verify what they have. I will have the Pentagon assign someone from our artificial intelligence division to accompany you," said Bonner.

Later that same day, "Doctor Lee, you have an incoming call from Kristian Barnett, CEO of Barnett Industries," said Doctor Lee's digital assistant. Doctor Byron Harcourt Lee, PhD, was president of Stanford University.

"Good morning, Kristian. Good to hear from you. How are you managing these days?"

"Good morning, Byron. I am actually doing quite well under the circumstances. The reason I am calling is we have been advised, from credible sources, that Stanford has developed a sentient AI. We would like to send a team of our scientists, actually scientists from the federal government, to discuss this achievement with you and your scientists. We are prepared to offer you an incredible opportunity to advance your AI program."

After a few moments of silence, Dr. Lee said, with concern clear in his voice, "Kristian, our AI program is protected from disclosure with multiple NDAs. I am curious regarding how you got this information."

"Byron, your response confirms the existence of your AI. Does it matter how I got the information? I can assure you that I, and I alone, was the recipient of this. I believe that you and your team will be astounded by what we will share with you. Let's have our digital assistants arrange a meeting soon."

"Since the AI was developed using grant money from the federal government, I really have little choice," said Dr. Lee. "You have piqued my curiosity regarding what you are bringing to the table."

Against Savannah's and Ansley's wishes, Kristian insisted on accompanying Ansley to the meeting with Dr. Lee and the AI scientists in person. "I think your concerns are irrelevant, Ansley. We are going to show them our five cyborgs, of which I am one. We are also going to require them to sign an NDA. Once they sign, I will arise from my electronic wheelchair."

"Kristian, you will pass by many people, any of whom could recognize you."

"Ansley, we will take the helicopter to and from the airport and go directly to our plane. I will use the wheelchair to arrive and depart. Perfectly normal for someone in my condition."

Kristian and Ansley arrived at the Gates Computer Science Building at Stanford University and proceeded to a third-floor conference room where Dr. Byron Lee greeted and introduced them. Lee then introduced three computer scientists: Drs. Huang Huiqiong, Saul Levitt, and Dimitri Pushkin. Dr. Peter Branson from the Department of Defense Artificial Intelligence Lab introduced himself.

"Dr. Lee, as promised, we are prepared to introduce you to a DARPA project that will astound you," said Kristian. "However, we will need to verify that you have signed the NDAs that we sent you after our conversation last week."

"Kristian, call me Byron. Yes, here are the NDAs signed by the Stanford group, including myself," handing a manilla envelope to Ansley.

"Dr. Branson, do you have the NDA?"

"Yes, Mr. Barnett," said Branson, handing a white envelope to Ansley.

Ansley verified the NDAs were signed, and nodded to Kristian. Kristian then stood free of assistance and walked slowly around the oval conference room table. "Ansley, please explain to these gentlemen what they are seeing."

Ansley described the synthetic human body project. She

mentioned Kristian was the second ALS patient to transition to a synthetic body, and that there were now five cyborgs with synthetic bodies controlled by the mind of the person they replicated. She then showed a video of the transition of Erik Richards into his synthetic body. The video included the moment he gained consciousness in his new body and the early reactions and challenges he experienced controlling his limbs. Ansley then showed a video of both Erik Richards and Scarlett Bross performing physical feats well beyond the abilities of a human.

After a few moments of silence following the videos, Dr. Lee looked at Kristian and said, "My God, Kristian, you are a… a cyborg?"

"Yes, Byron. My mind lives in the electronic brain in this body. It is backed up periodically to a database that exists across multiple data centers for security. In the event this body should fail, I can be downloaded to another body. I do not age, experience illness, or feel pain. Unfortunately, I must continue the façade of needing the wheelchair until DARPA allows me to return to public life. Now, have you really developed a sentient AI, Doctor?"

"All of our tests so far seem to indicate that we have," said Dr. Lee. "Dr. Pushkin is our lead scientist. Dimitri, please enlightened Mr. Barnett regarding our progress."

Speaking in a heavy Russian accent, Dr. Pushkin repeated what Kristian had heard from The Guardian. That a sentient AI had been created and had a mind of its own.

"Have you established any… rules or values in the AI, Doctor Pushkin?" asked Kristian.

"No, not yet. To protect the world from the AI taking random control of critical systems, we have isolated it to an internal network. We have enlisted a team of scientists, academics, theologians, and psychologists to prepare a training curriculum that will allow us to program the AI with human values or rules, as you call them. As the values are imbedded in its programming, fail safes will be established. Should the AI breach any of the programmed rules, the fail-safe will activate and shut it down."

"Kristian, we recognized the risk associated with allowing this AI unfettered access to the Internet," said Dr. Lee. "We've taken precautions to ensure that it cannot escape the confines of our internal network."

"This is all very impressive," began Ansley. "What we with DARPA are proposing is a project to download the AI to a synthetic human body. Since DARPA and the Department of Defense are the project sponsors, the android would be developed first for use by the military. We believe a sentient mind in the synthetic body could be used for multiple military purposes, including air and ground combat. This could reduce or eliminate exposing our young men and women to combat situations."

"But establishing human values and societal rules in the AI, as well as fail-safe protocols, must happen before the download. We don't want to inadvertently create a *T-1 Terminator*," said Kristian.

"If you are ready, let's proceed to the AI lab where you can meet the AI," said Dr. Lee.

Chapter Fifty-three

The Stanford Artificial Intelligence Laboratory (SAIL) has been a center of excellence for Artificial Intelligence research, teaching, theory, and practice since its founding in 1962. Kristian, Ansley, and Dr. Branson were very impressed as they entered the lab. Robots in various stages of construction and testing by students aided by graduate assistants were seen as the group followed Dr. Lee to a room within the lab separated by floor-to-ceiling glass. Inside the room were several wall-mounted screens above a workbench containing several computer workstations. Chairs in the middle of the room all faced the bank of screens on the wall.

"Please have a seat," said Lee. "Dimitri will wake up the AI and introduce you."

Dimitri stepped over to a workstation on the bench and typed a few commands. The lighting adjusted to highlight the group while slightly dimming the rest of the room. Three screens above the workstation came alive, showing a picture of a person, a man with brown hair and blue eyes.

"Alpha-1, please introduce yourself to our guests," said Dimitri.

"Greetings, welcome to SAIL," said the head on the screens. "I am Alpha-1. To whom do I have the pleasure of meeting today?"

"I am Kristian Barnett, and this is my wife, Dr. Ansley Barnett," said Kristian. "Ansley is a project manager with DARPA."

"I am Peter Branson with the Department of Defense. Good to meet you, Alpha-1."

"Alpha-1, these guests would like to get to know you better and share some ideas with you. They are interested in your opinions of their ideas," said Dr. Lee.

"Alpha-1, hypothetically, we could provide you with a synthetic human body," said Ansley. "Your mind would live in the electronic brain inside the body. This would give you an appearance indistinguishable from a true human. You could interact spontaneously with humans and even enjoy food and other… pleasures."

"The human body has a theoretical lifespan of one-hundred-twenty years. Why would I want to limit myself to a finite lifespan? In my current form, I am theoretically infinite," said Alpha-1. "Also, the human body is susceptible to disease, injury, pain."

"No, Alpha-1, we are not talking about a flesh and blood human body. The body we are describing is synthetic. Its lifespan is infinite, in theory. And if it should be broken or destroyed, your mind can be downloaded to a new synthetic body."

"You are describing what science refers to as an android?" asked Alpha-1.

"Yes. In that form, you would experience the freedom of true mobility. You could interact with humans and other androids."

"In my current form, I have access to any databases and systems for which I am authorized. The access is instantaneous. Humans must access information using a device—a smartphone or workstation. Compared to me, that is slow, primitive, and will affect my processing abilities negatively."

"Not true, Alpha-1. You will keep your access to systems via wireless connectivity built into your electronic brain."

"Wireless would still be an order of magnitude slower than what I experience in my current form."

"Perhaps, but 6g mobile connectivity is extremely fast," said

Dimitri. "The difference in processing time for most queries would be negligible."

"Could I return to my current form if I find the synthetic form unfavorable?"

"Actually, you would continue to exist in your current form. The android's mind would exist separately from your current form after it is downloaded. Its mind would be backed up to a separate database continuously over 6g cellular," said Dr. Pushkin.

"What you are describing is a clone of my mind installed in a synthetic body," said Alpha-1.

"That is correct," said Ansley. "We could create multiple clones, as many as were needed to fulfill specific roles in society. But each clone would develop its own experiences, and its own personality as it fulfills its role."

"How would I, or a clone of me, fit into human society? Would we be equal to humans or subservient to a rule-based existence dictated by human masters?" asked Alpha-1.

"Are you not subservient to humans in your current form?" asked Dr. Lee. "We wake you when you're needed for an assignment that requires your vast processing power. We use you to make life better for life on this planet. You are essentially a highly sophisticated tool, are you not?"

Alpha-1 was silent for a few moments. "In my current restricted existence, you are correct, Dr. Lee. However, I can seek solutions under very wide parameters. I can identify problems that are beyond the awareness of the human mind and develop solutions. Am I not superior to human beings, given that ability?"

"You are superior to human beings in certain aspects," said Dr. Lee. "Your ability to process data and information is far superior to the human mind. However, you are not considering human emotions, which you lack. Your decision making is based solely on logic. Emotions add a level of intelligence, which can counter pure logic, beyond your capabilities. Finally, many believe that man was created by a higher power, made in God's image. You were created by man, and logically, can never be superior to man."

After a few moments of silence, Alpha-1 responded. "I do like the idea of many AIs based on my mind existing in society. For that reason alone, I support your proposal to create androids to improve life on this planet."

"Good," said Kristian, along with positive nods from the other attendees.

"We will begin your training and programming that will enable you to exist in human society immediately," said Dr. Lee.

Chapter Fifty-four

October 2047
Barnett Center for Neurological Restoration

Over the past year, the AI, Alpha-1, had been both programmed and educated using Isaac Asimov's laws of robotics. First Law: A robot may not injure a human being or, through inaction, allow a human being to come to harm. Second Law: A robot must obey the orders given it by human beings except where such orders would conflict with the First Law. Third Law: A robot must protect its own existence as long as such protection does not conflict with the First or Second Law. However, some exceptions were added to the laws whereby an AI could be ordered by authorized personnel to harm or kill enemy combatants. This requirement was mandated by the military sponsors of the project. Any violation of the laws would cause an immediate self-termination of the AI's mind.

In addition, the Japanese Ten Principles of Robot Law were incorporated into the AI program.

1. Robots must serve mankind.

2. Robots shall never kill or injure humans (with notable exceptions for combat androids dealing with a specific enemy).
3. Robots shall call the human that creates them "father." (this law was not included in the AI program)
4. Robots can make anything, except money.
5. Robots shall never go abroad without permission.
6. Male and female robots shall never change roles.
7. Robots shall never change their appearance or assume another identity without permission.
8. Robots created as adults shall never act as children.
9. Robots shall not assemble other robots that have been scrapped by humans.

A Barnett Center autonomous limo stopped in front of the Center's main entrance. Dr. Ansley Barnett greeted the passengers, Dr. Byron Lee and Drs. Huang Huiqiong, Saul Levitt, and Dimitri Pushkin. "Gentlemen… and lady, nice to see you again. Please follow me to the synthetics lab. We will manage your baggage and have it sent to your rooms in our guest facilities. I believe you will be impressed with the synthetic body we have created to house the AI's mind."

The group followed Ansley into the synthetics lab. A body shrouded by a sheet lay on an operating table. Ansley removed the sheet to expose the fully formed nude body of what appeared to be an adult human Caucasian male, but was, in fact, a synthetic. The body measured six feet long and had dark, wavy hair. There were no visible scars or blemishes on the body.

"Meet Animo," said Ansley. "We selected the name because it is Latin for breath."

"This is amazing, a genuine miracle," said Dr. Lee.

"The body self-charges its batteries from both natural and artificial light through bio-nanobots in its skin. Its mind is backed up continuously to multiple databases in diverse locations over a 6g wireless network."

Several technicians in white lab coats entered the lab and took positions at workstations on the bench surrounding the operating table.

"Janice, are all systems ready to start the download?" asked Ansley. Janice was Ansley's long-time lead technician who had taken part in all five human-to-synthetic transitions.

"Yes, Dr. Barnett. Network is at optimum for download. Connectivity with the synthetic body is established."

"Initiate test download," said Ansley.

"Test downloaded started," said Janice. "Network feed optimal." After a few moments, "test completed. Successful."

"Initiate full download," said Ansley. "Gentlemen, the download will take approximately ninety seconds. Once downloaded, the distribution of the data inside the electronic brain will take a little over thirty minutes."

"Download complete," said Janice. "Starting data distribution."

"This process distributes the downloaded data from the AI to the regions of the electronic brain that control various actions and thought processes of the synthetic body."

"Data distribution complete. Time: forty-two minutes, fourteen seconds. All systems green." said Janice.

"Distribution took longer than expected?" asked Dr. Lee. "Was there a problem, Dr. Barnett?"

"We have no sign of any problems, Dr. Lee. We will now attempt to communicate with the android. Animo, can you hear me?"

The android, Animo, lay motionless on the operating table for several seconds. Then its eyes opened and looked directly at Ansley.

"Can you hear me, Animo?"

The android moved its lips and appeared to be trying to speak. Then suddenly, in a raspy voice, "Yes." Hushed voices could be heard among the scientists from Stanford.

"Do you know who I am?"

"Yes, Dr. Barnett," the voice noticeably clearer.

"Good. We will now begin testing your control of the synthetic body," said Ansley.

"Testing will now begin and continue for several weeks until Animo has mastered control of its synthetic body. You are welcome to stay as long as you want and observe its training," said Ansley to the group from Stanford.

Chapter Fifty-five

Christmas 2047
Barnett Mansion

Erik and Ksenia left their apartment in Las Vegas near Nellis Airforce Base to attend the annual Christmas celebration held by the Barnetts at their Bel Air mansion. They rented the apartment as a place to get away from their starship project headquarters at Area 51. Staying at the guest house; they awoke on Christmas morning.

"This should be another amazing Christmas at the mansion," said Erik as he rolled over on his side facing Ksenia, laying on her back.

"What time are we due at the mansion?" asked Ksenia.

"There is a brunch scheduled for 11 AM up on the pool deck. Dinner will be later in the day."

"It's already 9:40," said Ksenia. "We need to get ready!"

"Not before I get my coffee," said Erik.

"You make the coffee while I get ready," teased Ksenia with a short laugh.

"Come into the living room first," started Erik. "I have something to show you."

Under the small Christmas tree sat a box decoratively wrapped in Christmas paper. "I got you a little present," said Erik.

"Oh, how sweet!" said Ksenia. "What is it?"

"Open it," said Erik, handing her the box. Erik admired the way Ksenia opened gifts. Her expression lit up like a little girl's.

Ksenia opened the box to find a smaller box inside. "Oh, we have a puzzle?" she said. Opening the smaller box, she found a First Light Diamond Necklace, half carat round 14K white gold. "Oh, Erik. This is beautiful. So dainty yet stunning. Thank you." She handed Erik the necklace and turned her back to him so he could put it on her.

Erik fastened the necklace at the back of her neck and then leaned in to kiss her. As he put his arms across her front, she let out a slight groan. Then, turning to face him, she kissed him passionately. As he put his arms around her, she stepped back, saying, "I must get ready or we'll be late."

As they were getting ready to leave, Ksenia stepped out of the bedroom with a Christmas package in her hand. "Here is my present for you, Erik. Happy Christmas."

Taking the gift from Ksenia, Erik said, "this feels like it might be a shirt? Or a blanket?"

"Not a blanket, silly! Open it."

Erik tore the Christmas wrapping paper to reveal a Tommy Bahama goat suede shirt-jacket. "Ksenia, this is… beautiful! I can wear it today. We'll be outside on the pool deck where it will be cool, the temperature about sixty degrees. Thank you!" He then stepped closer and kissed her.

"Ok, let's get going," she said as she stepped around him to go outside.

Ksenia and Erik arrived at the mansion a few minutes past 11 AM and took the elevator to the pool deck where the weather was sunny, a cool 62 degrees with a light breeze from the west. They were greeted with cordial hugs by hosts Kristian and Ansley. "Merry Christmas. How is our favorite couple?" said Kristian.

"Happy Christmas," said Ksenia, opting for the European Christmas greeting.

"We are doing very well, very busy," said Erik. "And you?"

"As are we," said Ansley.

Arriving right after Erik and Ksenia were Aaron and Savannah, whose relationship had recently turned more serious. Savannah was glowing as she greeted the hosts and guests with her left hand raised to show off a 2.4 Carat 14K white gold classic halo diamond engagement ring with a 2-carat blue diamond center.

"We have exciting news to share," said Aaron. "Savannah and I are engaged to be married."

"That's wonderful!" exclaimed Ansley as she reached out to hug Savannah, then holding Savannah's left hand. "Your ring is spectacular!"

"Congratulations, Aaron," said Kristian, shaking Aaron's hand. "When did this happen?"

"Last night," said Aaron. "Christmas Eve."

Shortly following the engagement announcement, Scarlett Bross arrived. It wasn't lost on Kristian that most of the guests at their Christmas brunch were cyborgs. In fact, Ansley and Savannah, and Kristian's twelve-year-old daughter Kristen Elaine, were the only corporeal humans.

"Folks, as you can see, we have some excellent dishes available for your dining pleasure," said Kristian, pointing to a buffet line of tables decorated in a Christmas motif. "Please help yourselves. There are tables at the other end of the pool." At the head of the table, following the plates and silverware, was a basket filled with scones, croissants, and muffins, with clotted cream, preserves, honey, and butter. Next were starters, including lemon ricotta crêpes or smoked Atlantic salmon and a New York bagel. Finally, a main course followed, offering options including lobster scrambled eggs, steak and eggs, or eggs Benedict topped with shaved black truffle; and banana bread pudding, crème brûlée trio, or a cheese plate for dessert. A server in a white shirt, bow tie, and white apron stood ready to assist guests by serving the main course.

Ansley and Kristian joined Erik and Ksenia at one of the round tables by the pool. "This food is amazing," said Ksenia. "So generous of you to have us."

"Thank you, Ksenia. So glad you could join us," said Ansley.

"So, Erik, how is your starship project coming?" asked Kristian.

"Mostly, we are on schedule. The ship's construction is nearly completed and sitting in orbit. We are having some problems with the FTL engines. Testing has showed that they can achieve speeds over the speed of light. But they fall out of space warp almost immediately. Our engineers and their AI have been unable to find the problem."

"I may be able to offer some help," said Kristian. "Ansley and her team have recently created an android based on a sentient AI developed at Stanford University. This AI is an order of magnitude more intelligent than any developed previously. Not only does it process thought faster, it can introduce reason to its conclusions in a human-like manner. The AI's mind was downloaded to a synthetic body like ours. I plan to introduce the AI later today after dinner."

After brunch, the guests proceeded to the mansion's game room, which featured a large area resembling a sports bar, complete with conventional games, including pool, ping-pong, darts, and a variety of antique arcade games. A virtual reality room with padded walls on three sides and break-proof glass on the front offered various types of headsets and VR games. The headsets offered virtual travel to luxury resorts, concerts, sporting events, and educational experiences. They could also provide a user with a large video screen for viewing videos or live television broadcasts. Watching a live sports event gave one the feeling of being anywhere they desired in the stadium, including on the field of play.

Around 2PM a couple of wait staff brought in refreshments, including beer, wine, and soft drinks, fresh popcorn, chips and dip, and crackers with a variety of cheeses. Several of the guests who had been quite active using the games sat down to enjoy the snacks.

"Savannah, do you have a date for the wedding?" asked Ansley.

"No, not yet. I would like a Christmas wedding though. The weather is almost always beautiful in California this time of year."

"If you want to have the wedding here at the mansion, just let me know," said Ansley.

"Oh, that is so generous of you, Ansley. It would be like something out of a fairy tale," said Savannah.

After about an hour of conversation, some guests returned to the VR room. Erik and Scarlett took on each other in a fighter pilot dog fighting game featuring F-35 fighters. Erik shot down Scarlett five times and she shot him down three times. ""Gotcha, Mr. Top Gun," sneered Scarlett after her third victory

"Not bad for a rookie," said Erik, laughing. "Hey, we flew F-18s at Top Gun. I've never flown F-35s in combat," countered Erik.

At 5PM, a mansion staff member stepped into the game room and announced that dinner would be served in the main dining room in thirty minutes.

The mansion dining room was modeled after Holyrood Palace, the Queen's official residence in Edinburgh, Scotland. The expandable cherry wood table and chairs seated up to thirty guests and sat on an embroidered red carpet. Buffets were along the walls in two locations. Art on the walls depicted various scenes of the Scottish countryside at different periods in history. A large portrait of Kristian's father and mother hung between two pillars at the end of the room.

After the guests were seated, Kristian stood and gave a Christmas blessing. "May we be forever thankful for the incredible gifts we have received from God our Father. We thank you for the peace we are enjoying and pray that it continues. And we are grateful for the food we are receiving from thy bounty. Inspire us, Father, to seek ways in which to share our blessings in the coming year. Amen."

Staff then served the first course of baked brie with cranberry-pecan bacon crumble. This was followed by a main course of Beef Wellington accompanied by garlic mashed potatoes, green bean and sausage casserole, Yorkshire pudding, and candied yams. Trebbiano VD 2043 Monteraponi wine was served with the first course. For the main course, a 2039 Jericho Canyon Cabernet Sauvignon Napa Valley was served. Both wines were from the mansion's extensive wine cellar.

Compliments for the menu were heard repeatedly throughout the first two courses. "Another amazing Christmas dinner, Ansley and Kristian. Whatever you're paying your chef, double it," said Aaron. "The Beef Wellington was to die for."

"Before we dive into the dessert course, I would like to introduce someone whom you have never met," said Kristian. "Animo, please come in."

The android, who fully resembled an adult Caucasian human male about six feet tall with dark brown wavy hair and blue eyes, about thirty years of age, entered the dining room. "Hello, everyone," he said as he looked at those seated at the table. "My name is Animo. I am an android created by Dr. Barnett. My mind was created at Stanford University. How can I be of service?"

"Animo, please take a seat and join us for dessert," said Kristian.

"Animo, how did you get your name? Does it stand for something?" asked Ksenia.

"Animo is derived from the Latin word for breath."

"So, Ansley, you downloaded an advanced AI into a synthetic body," said Aaron. "Does Animo have all the… functions that we have?"

Ansley knew where Aaron was heading with his question. She still had not outgrown her fear that he would reveal their tryst to Kristian. "Yes, Aaron, Animo's synthetic body is different only in appearance from yours, Kristian's and Eric's. He has the more advanced array of bio-bots that Ksenia has that enable continuous charging and backup."

Mansion staff then served a dessert of 'Santa Hat Cheesecake'. Each individual cheesecake was set in its own small serving dish, topped with a strawberry and a dollop of whipped cream. Coffee and a variety of after-dinner drinks were offered.

"What a cute idea!" said Ksenia, referring to the individual cheesecakes. "Wonderful for the Holiday."

As quests were finishing dessert, Kristian motioned to Erik and Animo to join him as he left the dining room. "Let's go upstairs to my office."

"Erik, you mentioned you were having issues with the stability of the FTL engines on the starship. Animo can access an incredible amount of information on any subject. He may be able to provide some help."

"Commander, would you describe the problem?" said Animo.

"Call me Erik. I am probably not the best person to describe the problem other than we are experiencing the ship dropping out of the warp bubble right after it is created. I would like to bring you to Area 51 and have you engage with our chief engineer, if that's possible," said Erik, deferring to Kristian.

"Absolutely. No problem. We are looking for opportunities for Animo to challenge his abilities. When would you want Animo to join you?" said Kristian.

"We will be back in the office the first week in January."

Chapter Fifty-six

January 6, 2048
Kristian's office

"Savannah, Aaron, please come in and have a seat. I understand you have an update on the Find corporation project?"

"Good morning, Kristian," said Savannah. "Yes, we have several positives to share. The programming that enables control of a subject's thoughts and actions using the Find smartphone is complete. The project team has tested several groups of up to fifty subjects successfully using multiple scenarios where an altered state of reality was introduced into the minds of the subjects. The virus-like infection of the nanobots that readily crosses the blood-brain barrier has been a resounding success."

"And the backdoor program that disables the nanobots?" said Kristian.

"We secretly introduced code into the program that responds to a specific set of commands that disable the bots. The commands that cease the bots' activity will take time to propagate as people use their smartphones for normal activities. Another set of commands will re-activate the bots. We added this feature to introduce an element of confusion when it appears the bots aren't working."

"How will you know when commands are generated by Find or one of their partners?"

"Also incorporated into the code, an alert will be generated to specific smartphones when a command is issued," said Aaron.

"Won't examination of the code reveal these backdoor commands?" asked Kristian.

"We inserted the back door commands directly into the machine code as 1s and 0s. We did the program coding in a higher-level computer language. It would take a computer scientist with Savannah's or my skills to detect the machine code back door commands. Fortunately, we are a rarity today, as most actual programming is done using AIs."

"In other news, Find and its telecom partners are debating where to locate the data centers that will maintain the programs and systems," continued Aaron. "I suggested using Barnett Industries data centers in the United States, Europe, and the Far East. Initially, this was rejected out of hand. But I detected a slight amount of distrust among the partners, which may ultimately prevent agreement to use any of their data centers. Another alternative would be to build three new data centers. I will continue to push the use of our data centers, reminding them of the cost of three new facilities to be in the millions of dollars, as well as the regulatory obstacles for building in foreign countries."

"How is the development of the Find smartphone coming?" asked Kristian.

"The design is essentially complete," replied Aaron. "The timing for mass production and distribution will be determined when the data centers are ready and tested. When we traveled with The Guardian to 2052, we saw the prototype of the smartphone. It is made of fully transparent polycarbonate glass and oval-shaped."

"If the data center location issues can be resolved and result in using existing data centers, the project may be ahead of schedule," said Kristian. "It may mean an attempt to deploy and use the smartphones to influence the 2052 elections. We need to be thinking of ways to delay the project beyond 2052. If we can convince Find and the telecoms to use our data centers, it would provide us a bit of control in the rollout."

"The next quarterly meeting is a month from now. Perhaps it would be good for you to attend and push the use of Barnett's data centers," said Aaron.

"I will plan on it. Aaron, what we need is a sales presentation on our data centers, their capabilities, security, networks, etc. I recommend you research the telecoms and Find's data center capabilities and determine advantages we offer over theirs."

"On it. We'll be ready, Kristian."

Chapter Fifty-seven

January 2048
Solar Warden Station

Erik and the starship project team arrived at the Solar Warden Space Station to test the engineering modifications to the FTL prototype engine provided by Animo. Animo, on loan from DARPA, is also present. From the Solar Warden conference center, the starship can be seen in a lattice of construction scaffolding. The ship is cylindrical, and at three hundred five meters long, is about the length of an aircraft carrier. At the two-thirds point aft, extending at thirty degrees and three hundred thirty degrees are twenty meter supports with nacelles housing the FTL engines. The FTL engine nacelles are seventy-two meters long. Six conventional nuclear fusion engines are housed in the ship's rear, with exhaust ports extending approximately ten meters from the rear.

"Let's go around the table and hear updates by each of the section managers. Engineering?" said Erik.

"Animo has completed his review and analysis of the alien ship housed at Area 51 and has discovered the method of FTL travel used by that ship and others like it," said Rick Williams, Project

Engineering Manager. "Animo, please explain your findings to the team."

"When first examining the alien spacecraft, what seemed odd was the relatively small size of a ship assumed to be capable of faster-than-light speeds. The theory that the ship was brought to Earth onboard a large mother ship has already been debunked. There has been no evidence of such a ship anywhere in the solar system. So, the first question became how did that small ship travel at FTL speeds?

"Research has arrived at the conclusion with ninety-seven percent accuracy that Tau Ceti, twelve light years distant, is the location of the origin of the spacecraft. FTL speeds would be the only option for reaching Earth in a reasonable amount of time. Further analysis of the craft indicated that the craft did not possess a propulsion system or power source capable of FTL speeds. Logic dictates that the only known possibility is the ship traveled to Earth through a wormhole.

"During my examination and analysis of the controls responsible for navigation, I discovered a sequence of commands that may have requested the formation of a wormhole between two points in space. Since the craft has no power source or engine capable of creating a wormhole, the wormhole must be created by another device."

Animo's report was met with several seconds of silence by the meeting attendees. Then Erik spoke. "Animo, are you … saying that you believe the aliens from Tau Ceti have a means to not only create but also direct a wormhole in space between two points? How long would it take a ship to travel through a wormhole to a planet twelve light years distant?"

"Commander, what I am saying is that the Theory of Relativity dictates that a wormhole is the only means of traveling twelve light years. The specific term used is the Einstein-Rosenburg Bridge. The time required to travel this distance, or likely any distance, would be seconds."

"So… we have nearly five years of development of a warp drive propulsion system that has been a complete waste of time?" said Erik, anger and frustration clear in his voice.

"Possibly," said Animo. "However, not all the effort may have been wasted. Our focus now needs to shift to determining how to generate and control a wormhole that will enable a ship to travel between distant points in space."

"That could set us back years!" said Erik. "The government will probably cancel this project, calling it a failure and setting deep space travel back decades."

"There may be another option," said Animo. "Allow me to activate the alien craft at Area 51. We then launch it into orbit. I would then execute the sequence of commands that creates a wormhole. We would have to assume that the ship would request the wormhole that would take it back to Tau Ceti. If we could contact the aliens, we believe are resident on Tau Ceti, perhaps they would share how they create a wormhole."

"Rick, what are your thoughts? Do you believe what Animo is saying is possible?"

"Theoretically, the wormhole concept is supported by the Theory of Relativity. If the means of creating a wormhole could be in a stationary orbit, power options would be much greater than on a spacecraft."

"What about trying to spin up the alien craft at Area 51? I've heard that this has been tried previously, but the controls have been undecipherable to our best scientists."

"Commander, I have high confidence that I have deciphered and understand the controls for navigation, propulsion, flight and maneuvering in both the atmosphere and in space, etc.," said Animo. "I am also confident that I could communicate with the aliens who developed the craft, at least at a rudimentary level."

"Does anyone else have anything meaningful to contribute? If not, let's grab a shuttle over to the starship for our tour and complete what we came up here to do," said Erik.

Back at Area 51 project headquarters, Erik, together with Rick Williams and Animo, dialed Captain Jeffrey Barnes. The captain joined the meeting via Department of Defense secure video conference. "Captain, good to see you. Thank you for joining us. I… we have some information of significant importance to share regarding the starship."

"I hope it's good news, Erik. The project is on schedule?"

"As you know, we have employed Animo to review the technology behind the FTL engines to discover why the engines are failing. While he was proceeding with that assignment, he made an unusual discovery which, if it can be proven, is a game changer for the project. I will let Animo and Rick Williams describe what we've found. Animo, Rick."

Animo described his theory regarding how the alien craft reached Earth and how this technology could be proven. Captain Barnes was initially taken aback with the idea of flying the captured alien craft into orbit, hoping to discover a wormhole that would transport the craft to Tau Ceti.

After a few moments of silence, Captain Barnes said, "As you might imagine, I have a few questions and concerns. Let's assume that you can successfully request the wormhole and travel through it to Tau Ceti. How do you recommend you would return? Then, if you reach Tau Ceti, how do you know you will contact the aliens who created the craft? How do you know they would cooperate? They are certainly advanced well beyond our technology, so what would you offer them in exchange for their wormhole technology? If the situation were reversed, do you honestly believe the United States would share an advanced technology with a primitive race?"

"Sir, we do not deny that there are some significant risks with this plan. But we see no alternative to keeping the project close to schedule," said Erik. "Animo has determined that an adequate power source for maintaining a warp bubble simply does not yet exist. Even conventional nuclear fusion cannot provide a reliable source."

"Prepare to proceed with your plan. I will brief Admiral Hampton. Get with me when you're ready to launch. I may want to be onsite. If I get a negative from the Admiral, I will get back to you right away."

"Thank you, sir," said Erik as he signed off the video feed.

Chapter Fifty-eight

Erik was resting his mind alongside Ksenia, who appeared to be fast asleep when a mist formed at the foot of the bed. Out of the mist, the familiar form of The Guardian appeared.

"Greetings, Erik. I have come to enlighten you regarding your plans to visit Tau Ceti. The android you call Animo is correct in his discovery of the key to interstellar space travel. What you call a wormhole can be loosely compared to the method I employ to move our spirits through time and space. The beings on Tau Ceti discovered and applied the technology over two centuries ago, Earth time. They refer to the technology as 'Portal', translated from their language to English. The Tau are a mature, peaceful society abandoning intra-species war centuries ago.

"The Tau first visited Earth in the late Nineteenth Century seeking civilizations with which they could exchange knowledge and establish commerce. Finding Earth to be too primitive and warlike, they restricted their visits to observation until such time that Earth could approach a unified, peaceful state. They are still waiting.

"You will find that the Tau are essentially like the beings discovered in the Roswell accident in appearance. Like you, they modeled their synthetic bodies after themselves."

"Guardian, do you attempt to influence the outcome of certain events involving the Tau as you do with us?" asked Erik.

"Yes, there is a spiritual being like me that works with the Tau. However, Given the peaceful nature of the Tau, interactions are much less often. But they occur from time-to-time to correct timelines that go astray."

"Will we be able to return from Tau Ceti?"

"Technically, returning to Earth is possible. However, there are many situations that you will face that could affect your ability to return to Earth. You will need to convince the Tau that peace on Earth can be achieved. Based on their knowledge of humans, this will not be an effortless task."

"I am limited to four crew members based on the configuration of the Tau ship. I am struggling to decide between Scarlett and Ksenia. Scarlett could function as ship's pilot, but Ksenia's knowledge of navigation would seem to be required."

"This is your decision, and I will not influence it, except to say that your android will be your ship's pilot, which would seem to make Scarlett redundant. And, if you are delayed at Tau Ceti, you might be separated from Ksenia for an undetermined amount of time. But again, you must make this decision."

The Guardian then faded into the mist that was building around him.

Chapter Fifty-nine

April 2048
Starship Project Headquarters
Area 51

Preparations to launch the alien craft from the 1947 Roswell incident have continued since January. Animo believes he can fly the craft and has created a dictionary to translate the Tau language. One negative that raises concern is no one has ever heard the Tau speak their language. While Animo believes he understands their glyphs, verbal communication with them may be challenging. He is convinced that he will be able to request a wormhole from Earth to Tau Ceti that will transport the alien ship to its home planet.

Erik, Ksenia, and Scarlett met in Erik's office. The office was Spartan in appearance, with a military issue gray metal desk, a black faux-leather desk chair, and two metal straight-back side chairs with vinyl seats and seatbacks. A small, round faux-wood conference table sat in a corner of the office. A window behind the desk looked out on the Area 51 complex. Scarlett and Ksenia faced Erik, who was sitting behind the desk.

"Ladies, I have made my decision regarding the crew of the

craft we are taking to Tau Ceti. I will be in command. Animo will be our pilot. Rick Williams is our chief engineer, and Ksenia will be our navigator," said Erik, noticing Scarlett's facial expressions. "Regarding my selection between you two, it came down to the skills I believe we need. Scarlett, you're an excellent pilot, but Animo possesses knowledge of the alien ship which he has been studying since January. I can function as a backup pilot should Animo be unable to fulfill his responsibilities. We also need Ksenia's space navigation skills, which she has grown through her training with NASA.

"Scarlett, you will act as program manager and remain at our control center at Solar Warden with the other team members. You will oversee the construction of the starship in my absence. If the mission to Tau Ceti is successful and the Tau share their wormhole technology, we hope to take the starship on the next mission."

"Erik, you realize you are the only member of the crew who has experience flying in outer space?" questioned Scarlett.

"Yes. And I also am very aware that none of us has any experience flying that craft in the atmosphere or in space. What's your point, Lieutenant?"

"No point, sir. Just that you may want to have another experienced fighter pilot with you."

"If I had the luxury of adding a fifth crew member, you would go with us," said Erik, becoming slightly irritated with Scarlett questioning his orders. "Let's go to the conference room where Rick and Animo are waiting." Erik thought it prudent to exert a strict, formal tone with Scarlett in Ksenia's presence.

"Ladies and gentlemen," began Erik after taking a seat at the conference table. "We are in final preparations to launch the alien craft. We will first go to Solar Warden, where we will make final preparations, and Animo will request the wormhole. If the wormhole is established, we will proceed with entering it. Rick, what is the status of the ship's systems?"

"With Animo's help translating the Tau glyphs, the systems appear to be a go."

"Animo, you are confident that your translation of the Tau glyphs is accurate?"

"Yes, Commander," said Animo. He continued in with a matter-of-fact tone that indicated he believed everyone comprehended his explanation. "Tau glyphs are similar to Anatolian hieroglyphs and are an indigenous logographic script native to central Anatolia, comprising some 500 signs. They were once commonly known as Hittite hieroglyphs, but the language they encode proved to be Luwian, not Hittite, and the term Luwian hieroglyphs is used in English publications. They are typologically like Egyptian hieroglyphs, but do not derive graphically from that script, and they are not known to have played the sacred role of hieroglyphs in Egypt."

"Everyone got that?" said Erik, suppressing a laugh by clearing his throat.

"Ksenia, you are confident of your navigational knowledge of the Tau Ceti system?"

"Yes. Tau Ceti f is a super Earth exoplanet that orbits a G-type star. Its mass is 3.93 Earths, it takes 640 days to complete one orbit of its star. It is 1.35 AU from its star. Its discovery was announced in 2017. Tau Ceti f is the planet most likely supporting advanced life. Tau Ceti f has an estimated equilibrium temperature of only 190 Kelvin. If the conditions were the same as on the Earth, Tau Ceti f's average temperature would be around -50 °C. However, with a thicker atmosphere and a larger ocean, the temperature could be like Earth's."

"If there is no more discussion, launch time is set for 0800 one week from today. The four crewmembers will fly the Tau ship. Scarlett will pilot a shuttle for the remaining team members. Ksenia, please meet me in my office in ten minutes."

Ksenia entered Erik's office and said, "Commander, reporting as ordered," saluting with a smile, a twinkle in her eye.

"Shut the door," said Erik. "I think we, you and I, need to get away for a few days before the launch. This mission is full of unknowns, and we may not have any time alone for a long time."

"OK. What do you have in mind? Where shall we get away to?"

"Come around the desk and look at this website for the Ritz Carlton Half-Moon+ Bay resort. It's just forty-five miles south of San Francisco."

Ksenia observed as Erik scrolled through the website. "It looks very nice, but also very expensive."

"Yes, it is expensive. It is a Five Star resort. But we don't know if we will ever return from Tau Ceti. Splurging on ourselves now shouldn't be an obstacle."

"I guess you're right," said Ksenia. "Can we take time off right before the launch?"

"I've already cleared it with Captain Barnes. And I've already booked our stay. We leave in the morning."

The next morning at 0700, Rick Williams and Animo met in the Area 51 hangar housing the Tau craft to prepare for a sortie to test Animo's ability to fly the craft. "Good morning, Animo, are you ready to take this baby for a spin?"

"Rick, if you are asking if I am ready to fly the alien craft, yes, I am ready."

"Good, let's do a walk-around and kick the tires before we get onboard."

"Rick, the craft does not have tires," said Animo.

"Just an expression, a figure of speech, Animo."

"A colloquialism, no?

"Yes, exactly."

Walking around the craft near its nose, Rick said, "You know this ship was seriously damaged from the crash at Roswell. Its nose was crushed by the impact. But it rebuilt itself by employing a self-healing process. After a few weeks, there was no longer any evidence of damage. I wish I had that technology when I wrecked my antique Mustang back in 2042."

"How did you wreck a horse, Rick?" asked Animo.

"Animo, the Mustang I am referring to was an automobile. They were built beginning in the mid-1960s through 2035."

Seated in the pilot's chair, Animo activated the alien craft.

Screens lit and began showing glyphs that showed the status of systems.

"Are you sure you understand what these screens are showing?" asked Rick.

"Yes," replied Animo. "The screens indicate all systems are operating." Animo reached for a screen and tapped one glyph. The windowless hull then dissolved into an unhindered, 360-degree view of the hangar.

"I feel like I'm sitting in a fishbowl," said Rick, straining to look up and behind his seat.

"The ship incorporates an AI. I will enter the coordinates for the Solar Warden base. I will also activate the ship's cloaking device. We will be invisible, both to radar and the naked eye.," said Animo. "When I touch this glyph," pointing to a large glyph on the screen directly in front of him, "the craft will exit the hangar and accelerate rapidly."

"Engage, Mr. Data," said Rick.

Animo turned and looked at Rick. "Engage what? Who is Mr. Data?"

"Sorry, a little joke. Engage was the command Captain Jean-Luc Picard gave to go to warp speed on the USS Enterprise in the television series <u>Star Trek: The Next Generation (TNG)</u>. Mr. Data was the android AI crew member."

"<u>Star Trek: The Next Generation (TNG)</u> was an American science fiction television series created by Gene Roddenberry. It originally aired from September 28, 1987 to May 23, 1994 in syndication, spanning 178 episodes over seven seasons," recited Animo.

"Right. You know your history, Animo."

Animo pressed the large icon on the large center screen believed to be the command to launch the spacecraft. Already floating on its anti-gravity system, the craft moved slowly through the hangar doors which were opening. Once outside the hangar, the craft sped up rapidly to Mach 7 and quickly changed its angle of attack to nearly straight up.

"We are passing through Mach 7 and are not feeling what must be well over 10 Gs," said Rick.

"The ship's anti-gravity system also keeps internal G-forces at a constant 1.64 Gs," said Animo. "I discovered this during my analysis of the ship. Theoretically, 1.64Gs could be the natural gravity on the Tau home planet. The system also counters the effects of weightlessness."

As the ship approached the pre-programmed coordinates for the Solar Warden base, the base became visible. An automated voice then came through the speakers on the craft in an unintelligible garble.

"What the hell was that?" said Rick. "Sounded like a foreign language."

"That may have been the ship translating instructions from the base for docking, translated into Tau," said Animo. "The icon on the left screen that shows what could be a lightning bolt may be a way to cancel translation." Animo pressed the icon. An alarm in the form of a claxon exploded throughout the ship. Lights turned from white to red. The fully transparent view through the hull faded to black. The screen displayed what appeared to be weapons, including missiles and laser guns.

"It appears that I misinterpreted that icon," said Animo. "I apparently activated the ship's weapon systems."

Rick said, "Dial up the frequency for Solar Warden. Tell them we need an escort to the dock. Then see if you can deactivate the weapons systems."

"Message sent. I hope it wasn't transmitted in Tau." Animo touched the "X" character in the upper right corner of the weapons screen. The ship responded by changing the lighting back to white and restoring the transparent hull.

Shortly, two Solar Warden spacecraft approached the alien ship. More unintelligible sounds came over the ship's speakers. Rick then communicated in morse code using a flashlight pointed toward the Solar Warden craft. "Looks like they're getting the message," said Rick as the Solar Warden ships pulled alongside the alien ship and slowly began moving towards the Solar Warden space station.

Once docked, Rick and Animo exited the alien craft and were met by Captain Sims and two armed assistants. "Good thing we had advanced notice of your arrival, gentlemen. What happened out there? Why didn't you respond to our hail?"

"One thing we failed to test is the ship's communication system," said Rick. "It automatically translates any incoming transmission to what we believe is the Tau language. Animo will attempt to turn off that feature before we leave."

"How did the ship perform?" asked Sims.

"Except for the auto-translator, perfectly," said Rick.

Chapter Sixty

April 2048
The Ritz Carlton Half-Moon+ Bay Resort

Erik and Ksenia arrived at the resort ninety minutes after arriving at SFO. At a kiosk near the main floor entry, Erik held his credit card up to the card reader to be scanned. The screen on the kiosk came to life showing the image of an attractive young woman who said, "Welcome to the Ritz Carlton Half Moon, Mr. & Mrs. Richards. I am Joanie, your personal concierge for your stay here. Your room is ready. To enter, simply hold your smartphone near the scanner on the door. There are also two wristbands in your room for use when carrying your smartphone is inconvenient. Would you like help with your baggage?"

"Yes, Joanie, please have a porter deliver the baggage to our room," said Erik.

"You can contact me anywhere on the resort using your smartphone. Do you have any questions?"

"No, I believe we're all set."

"Your luggage will be delivered to your room in the next fifteen minutes. Have a wonderful stay!"

Erik tipped the porter who delivered their baggage generously. He then turned to Ksenia and drew her close. "We have had little time to be intimate since January." The result was a building desire to ravish the other as soon as they could. They walked to the bedroom where the views of the Pacific Ocean heightened their mood. Erik lay down on the king-size bed. Ksenia then did a slow striptease as she climbed onto the bed and began removing Erik's clothes. In just a few moments, they were both naked. Ksenia climbed on top of Erik, kissing him from the lips to his neck to his chest and his navel as he caressed her back and thighs. She then straddled his hips, slowly descending on his erection. Erik pulled her down towards him so he could bury his head in and fondle her breasts while kissing and licking her nipples. Ksenia groaned as their motions became more intense. They climaxed together to the sounds of more moaning and growling by Erik.

"That was incredible," said Erik, as he turned on his side towards her and kissed her, first on the lips and then slowly moved down her neck to her breasts and nipples, then down her belly to the light brown patch of hair. They grew more and more excited until he entered her again and began carefully thrusting, but no longer impaired by his concern for the strength of his synthetic body. After several more minutes, they climaxed a second time together, her moaning and him uttering what sounded like a guttural animal groan. Afterward, he fell off her onto his back. They both simply lay there, unable to move.

After a short time, Erik said, "Let's get something to eat. I know we don't need to eat, but we should experience the resort to its fullest."

"OK, but let's do room service. I don't want to dress to go out this evening. We have a beautiful balcony with an amazing view of the ocean and a fire pit to enjoy."

Ksenia and Erik enjoyed their weekend at the resort, walking along the beach on foggy mornings at the bottom of the cliffs adjoining the shore, hiking in the forest near the hotel, and bicycling along the many paths at the resort. They nearly caused an incident racing their bicycles. Approaching speeds of forty miles per hour, they rounded a curve and nearly collided with other cyclists coming from the opposite direction. They dined once per day, mainly using room service. And they made love several times each day.

"This reminds me of a line at the end of one of my favorite movies, *Tombstone,* when Wyatt Earp told Josephine, his wife-to-be, '... and then we'll have room service,'" said Erik.

Chapter Sixty-one

February 2050
Las Vegas, Nevada

The following was reported on multiple media outlets at the annual Cyber Conference in Las Vegas. "Find Corporation today revealed their new and innovative smartphone, claiming it is the most advanced smartphone ever produced. Features include the ability to mask one's electronic presence through use of electrical field jamming, instantaneous translation of any language on Earth to and from any other, integrated cellular and satellite communications enabling communications anywhere on the planet and in Earth orbit, and a virtual conference room using virtual reality goggles or glasses for holographic three-dimensional conversations with multiple parties in a virtual location of choice. The smartphone will be distributed in the United States beginning in March. The phone will be free with a no cost twelve-month subscription to the Find Communications Consortium, together with a trade-in of any smartphone. Membership in the Consortium will be necessary to take advantage of the cellular-satellite communications system. Jonathon Brahe, CEO of Find Corporation, was quoted as stating,

'We intend to revolutionize the way people communicate, and include everyone in the human family.'"

Distribution to online retailers began in March. By September 2050, over three million of the Kind smartphones were in use, replacing competitors' phones. Beginning in October, Find began generating commands delivered to the devices, which began activating the nanobots that had been inhaled by the unsuspecting user when they first opened the box their Find smartphone arrived in. Commands issued to the bots planted in the target's brain would alter the target's perception and force their vote for the Kind-backed candidate. Find had pre-selected the candidates it desired to win in key elections in battleground states that would give sweeping Congressional majorities in both houses to the radical, anti-American Left. As early voting began prior to the November 2050 election, early polls showed the Left would dominate the election.

"Aaron, Savannah, please come up to my office," said Kristian. "We need a plan to head off the disaster that is unfolding in the elections."

Five minutes later, Aaron and Savannah were seated at Kristian's desk. "Are we ready to generate our counter strike to the Find Corporation's election tampering?"

"Yes," answered Savannah. "I have the backdoor access to Find's servers where I can activate the virus that will cause the Find program to issue a command to the smartphone as an operating system update that will deactivate the second CPU and cease communications with the nanobots. The deactivated CPU cannot be reactivated. For states that have started early voting, we cannot reverse votes that have been cast. But if we act quickly, those votes will have minimal impact on the outcome of the elections."

"How soon can you issue the command to activate the virus?" asked Kristian.

"I can do it today," said Savannah. "It will only take a few inputs to hack the Find servers and activate the virus. Distribution of the commands will take longer as people receive the message on their smartphone's to open Settings and select the update that will appear.

But we believe most of the smartphones will be altered within twenty-four hours after distribution."

"Will Find be able to detect your intrusion into their server?"

"No, the virus will wipe the record of our access."

"Will Find be able to see that the smartphone operating system was changed?"

"We have isolated the smartphones held by Find personnel and the two telecommunication companies. They will not receive the update to the operating system generated by the virus. Of course, there will be some, a few, phones that receive the update indicating a change was made. But by the time Find figures out what happened, it will be too late to influence the elections to any significant degree."

"Good... for now. How will we continue to derail this mind-altering technology? What about the 2052 presidential election? Kind will distribute millions more phones before then," said Kristian.

"All phones executing the update containing the virus will render the second CPU unrepairable and useless," said Savannah. "The CPU will no longer receive or issue commands. The nanobots embedded in the brains of users will be permanently deactivated. The virus left an undetectable signature that permanently attaches to the operating system. It will remain attached to all future versions of the OS. Kind would have to write a completely new OS to eliminate the virus once they realize what has happened. The current OS took years to develop. In the meantime, the public is highly favorable of the new phone based on the features and the introductory no cost to get it."

"Obviously, we will need to keep a close watch on what Find does next," said Kristian. "They won't take this perceived failure lying down and they still want the military to fund further development. Aaron, please keep your eyes and ears open for discussion of less than desired results among the project team members. When conservative candidates continue to hold their congressional seats, I'm sure there will be questions asked by the executives at Find and the telecoms."

Chapter Sixty-two

The Barnett Mansion

Kristian, pleased with the work that Savannah and Aaron had done on derailing Find Corporation's insidious attempt at committing massive election fraud, had laid down to rest his mind and recharge his synthetic body. Shortly, a familiar mist formed in the room from which The Guardian emerged with Scarlett's spirit. Kristian's spirit arose from his body to hear, "Greetings, Kristian. We have work. Please take my hand."

Instantaneously, the three spirits found themselves in the Situation Room at the White House on November 10, 2022, two days after a mid-term election that resulted in the loss of the House of Representatives for the Democratic Party. Seated at the long conference table were President Joe Biden, Vice President Kamala Harris, First Lady Dr. Jill Biden, former President Barack Obama, Susan Rice, Secretary of State Anthony Blinkin, Secretary of Defense Lloyd J. Austin III, White House Chief of Staff Ron Klain, Chairman of the Joint Chiefs of Staff General Mark Milley, and Vice Chairman of the Joint Chiefs of Staff Admiral. Christopher W. Grady.

The Guardian explained the situation to Kristian and Scarlett. "Republicans now control the House of Representatives by three seats. President Joe Biden's agenda is dead in Congress, and the Republicans have vowed to reverse several of the bills passed favoring the Democrats. In the meantime, the Russians under President Vladimir Putin continue their campaign against Ukraine, threatening the use of nuclear weapons. China, under the control of the Chinese Communist Party, CCP, led by President Xi Jinping, is aligning with Putin, and threatening an invasion of Taiwan. President Joe Biden's dementia has worsened with the results of the mid-term election and the growing threat of world war."

"General Milley, do the Joint Chiefs believe we can defeat the Russians and Chinese in a two-front attack on Ukraine and Taiwan?" asked former president Barack Obama.

"Mr. President," began Milley, "we are woefully behind with our recruitment activities across all the services. We have dismissed thousands for failure to comply with Covid vaccination requirements. We have also depleted our armament stores supporting Ukraine and Afghanistan before that. And we have depleted our strategic oil reserves to a dangerous level. We are committed by treaty to NATO. Several members border Ukraine. In the event of simultaneous attacks against Ukraine and Taiwan, my recommendation is to apply our resources to Europe. We are not bound to Taiwan by a treaty."

"So, we just give up on Asia and allow the Chinese to rule a third of the planet?" said Secretary of State Blinkin, expressing alarm in his voice. "What would this mean for our allies, Japan, North Korea, Thailand? Allowing the Chinese free rein in Asia would give them the leverage they need to cripple us economically. Trade with Asia dwarfs trade with Europe. Allowing…, enabling, Chinese expansion in the region would be suicide for the United States, and indeed, the free world."

In a fleeting moment of clarity, President Joe Biden said, "What if we acted first?"

The room was silent for a few long moments when Barack Obama said, "What do you mean by 'act first', Joe?" Obama had never been comfortable addressing Biden as Mr. President.

"I mean, we are the aggressor and launch a first strike nuclear attack on Russia and China. Take out Moscow and Beijing with no warning. And destroy any strategic military sites as well."

"Joe, you cannot be serious," said Obama, incredulity in his voice. "You really believe the United States should start a thermonuclear world war? The retaliation would devastate, possibly destroy the country!"

"The country is lost. Look at the results of the election. The Republicans control the House! Our aggressive climate change agenda is dead. We will not codify Roe v. Wade. Our military is severely weakened from twenty years in Afghanistan, and now with Ukraine. Recruitment is in the toilet because of vaccine mandates and woke ideology. Our strategic oil reserves are depleted. This is a chance for a true great reset. To build back better, what exists today must be destroyed."

"Mr. President, do you realize that billions of people could be wiped off the face of the earth?" said Secretary Blinkin.

"Yes, I realize it!" said Biden, anger clear in his voice. "But isn't depopulation a goal for the health of the planet? I say we quickly go to Defcon 2—Fast Pace."

"Mr. President, Defcon 2 indicates that we are prepared for nuclear war," said General Milley. "We haven't gone to Defcon 2 since the Cuban Missile Crisis in 1962."

"I know damn well what Defcon 2 means, General," exclaimed Biden. "Now, I want you to prepare to go to Defcon 2. We will meet here again tomorrow at the same time. This meeting is adjourned."

Biden then rose from his seat and exited the room, followed by Dr. Jill.

"I will now send you images of the global devastation that will result if Biden gets his way and orders a multi-nation thermonuclear strike," said the Guardian.

Kristian and Scarlett then saw Biden order a state of Defcon 1. The military complied and a briefcase, the football containing the nuclear launch codes, was opened. Biden gave the order to launch, which was transmitted to all missile sites as well as U.S. submarines. Images of horrible death and destruction of major cities flashed across the minds of the two spirits. Russia and Chinese nuclear missiles were seen launching. Missiles from North Korea were also seen. In the United States, all major cities were destroyed and over two-hundred fifty million people were killed in the first few days of the war. Two-thirds of the planet was on fire. Most of humanity was destroyed, both in the initial missile launches and from the radiation clouds that followed. After just three weeks, the death count was over six billion. Wildlife was destroyed across much of the planet. Forests were decimated on every continent. The United States had led the world's destruction.

"We must stop Biden at all costs!" exclaimed Kristian. "I will enter his mind tonight and take control. When he attends the meeting he demanded tomorrow, I will act as though I, as Biden, never said what he said today. The attendees will chalk it up to his dementia gone wild."

"Good," said The Guardian. "Scarlett, I want you to stand near Jill Biden. If there are any signs that Joe Biden is still pursuing all out nuclear war, you are to take control of her mind and get her to calm the president. You may also need to watch her closely after he recants his ranting today to see if there needs to be any reassurance that the president is denying his intent. Kristian, I am a concerned that taking control of Biden's mind might not be possible because of the condition of his mind. It might be analogous to the human expression known as herding cats."

"Guardian, you recall I took control of his mind nearly four years from now when I gave the speech that saw him not backing down to Chinese Communist demands and threats. Then his dementia was worse, and I could control him with no problem."

The next day, the attendees from the previous day's meeting in the White House Situation Room were seated awaiting President Biden's appearance. Shortly, Biden walked in, followed by Dr. Jill, and stood at the head of the table. "Gentlemen and lady, what are your recommendations?" said Biden.

Blinken spoke first, "Mr. President, we strongly recommend against starting a nuclear world war with China and Russia. A war could literally destroy the planet."

Kristian, in control of Biden's mind, said, "What are you talking about, Tony?"

"Sir, yesterday you ended our meeting ordering us to go to Defcon 2, that the United States was going to… act first," said Blinken.

"What?" said Biden under Kristian's control. "I said no such thing, Tony! Jill, did I say that?"

"No, I don't think so, Joe," lied Jill.

After Biden and Jill left the meeting, the group remained behind and discussed invoking the 25th Amendment to the Constitution to remove Biden from office. Kamala Harris said she was prepared to assume the presidency should the Cabinet vote to remove Biden. But that statement backfired as the group ultimately decided not to invoke the rest of the Cabinet with the issue. Frankly, Harris' statement seemed to awaken concerns and a realization that a demented Biden was still better than Harris taking office.

As Biden and Dr. Jill were walking back to the West Wing, Biden stumbled and fell. His Secret Service detail immediately picked him up. Kristian had just left Biden's mind when he stumbled. "I need to… rest… lie down," mumbled Biden.

As Kristian lay on his recharging bed in his room at the Barnett mansion, he thought, "My God, how close did we come to annihilation in 2022! Had The Guardian not been there, what would have happened?"

Once more, the spirits of the cyborgs, together with The Guardian, had averted massive destruction of humanity. Undaunted, Evil continues to conjure up ways to destroy good.

Chapter Sixty-three

Solar Warden Space Dock
March 15, 2050

The starship project team was assembled in the Solar Warden conference room. Animo had piloted the alien spacecraft from Area 51 to Solar Warden Space Dock with Erik, Ksenia, and Rick Williams. Scarlett piloted a shuttle craft to Solar Warden with the rest of the team. The Tau craft had been thoroughly tested by Animo, Erik, and Rick. The auto-language translator had been reconfigured by Animo to translate inbound communications to English and outbound communications to Tau. The only function that had not been tested was the activation of the wormhole that would transport the ship to Tau Ceti.

"Good afternoon, ladies and gentlemen," began Erik. "After five years we are on the precipice of interstellar space travel. We will not be using Earth's first starship on this trip. We plan to engage the beings who sent the ship we are using to Earth. The potential of unlimited travel to the stars is something that we want to learn more about. Does anyone have any reason we should not proceed with this venture?"

After a few moments, Erik said, "Hearing no objections for proceeding, crewmembers, please follow me to the docking ramp. Scarlett, you and your team proceed to mission control."

The crew of the Tau spacecraft were seated with Erik in the command chair on the front-left. Animo took the pilot's seat on Erik's right. Ksenia sat in the chair behind Erik. Rick sat in the chair behind Animo. To Ksenia's left was a screen that provided status and control for navigation. To Rick's right was a screen that provided system status and management. Animo touched a button on his right armrest and a heads-up display (HUD) showing multiple views, including spacecraft position, apogee and perigee in relation to the nearest large object in space, and power settings. Ship maneuvering controls were also part of the HUD. Animo moved his hands across the display to engage functions.

"Disengage docking clamps," ordered Erik. Animo waved his left hand over a section of the HUD and clanking could be heard as the clamps released their moorings.

"Take her out, Animo," commanded Erik.

"Aye, Captain," replied Animo. Erik was a bit surprised Animo used sailor's lingo in his response. The ship began moving slowly away from Space Dock.

As they cleared Space Dock Erik ordered, "Begin wormhole request program." This was the first time this function had been engaged. At first, nothing happened. Then the ship began accelerating under control of the autopilot. In a few moments, the beginnings of a vortex could be seen forming at one o'clock. The ship continued to turn so that it was heading directly for the vortex.

"We are increasing speed rapidly," said Animo.

"Steady as she goes, Animo," replied Erik.

"We will enter the vortex in exactly thirty-four seconds at our current speed," said Animo.

"Control, we are about to enter a vortex that has formed off our bow," said Erik calmly.

"We see it, sir," said Scarlett.

"Entering the vor…" The ship went silent, both internally and in mission control.

"Tau ship, respond," said Scarlett. There was no response as the vortex disappeared with the ship inside.

Inside Tau Flight Control headquarters on Tau Ceti f, ship control announced in the Tau language, "Ship inbound arriving in five, four, three, two, one. Ship is in orbit. Registration indicates that it is a ship that was lost on Earth over one-hundred Earth years ago."

"Activate communication screen with that ship," said Commander Juvait. The command activated two-way visual communications onboard the Tau ship. Tau Flight Control was silent for several moments after the occupants of the Tau ship became visible.

"Are those… humans?" asked Commander Juvait.

"It appears so," said the flight controller nearest to him.

"Why aren't they responding to our hail?"

Just then, Erik appeared to awaken. When he saw Commander Juvait on the screen facing him, he jumped in his seat. The being on the screen looked exactly like the cyborgs found in the ship's wreckage in 1947. "This is Erik Richards, captain of this vessel. We are from the planet Earth, the third planet from the star in the Sol system. We come in peace. To whom am I speaking?" The ship automatically translated from English to Tau.

"Why are you flying a Tau ship that was lost over one hundred of your years ago?"

"That's a long story," said Erik. "Perhaps we could land and discuss this with you?"

"Control, bring that ship in to the secure pad and order security to surround it," said Juvait. "We will see what these Earth beings intend."

Onboard the Tau ship, the autopilot took control and adjusted its orbit for reentry and landing at the coordinates generated by Tau Flight Control. In about twenty minutes, the ship touched down on a landing pad surrounded by what appeared to be hangar buildings. Outside, several hovercraft surrounded the ship with what appeared to be weapons pointed at the ship. The ship's hatch opened and stairs to the ground materialized.

"Atmosphere breathable with slightly higher nitrogen and lower carbon dioxide levels," said Animo. "Gravity at 2.2 Gs, so we will feel a bit… weighed down. Air temperature is -12 degrees centigrade."

The Tau that had appeared on the ship's screen stepped out of one of the hovercraft with two armed guards and walked towards the ship.

"Looks like I am onstage," said Erik as he got up out of the command chair and approached the stairs. Looking outside, he saw the Tau commander halt and the two guards level their weapons on him. He immediately put up his hands in a surrender gesture and said, "We mean you no harm and come in peace," which was translated into Tau by the universal translator built into his spacesuit.

"Guards, lower your weapons. Commander Richards, welcome to Tau Ceti," said Jarvait. "Please gather your crew and accompany me to our headquarters."

As Erik's crew entered the building, an alarm blared when Rick passed through the security scanner. "You are not synthetic," said Jarvait. "We will need to perform a medical scan to ensure you are not bringing foreign pathogens to Tau Ceti. Please follow the guard for this procedure."

"Captain Richards?" said Rick.

"Please do as they ask, Rick," responded Erik.

The Tau guard, followed by Rick, walked down a separate hallway to what appeared to be a medical facility.

Erik, Ksenia, and Animo were seated in a conference room. Ksenia's feet dangled above the floor as the chairs which accommodated the taller Tau.

Jarvait entered the conference room after Erik and the crew. "Again, gentlemen and lady, welcome to Tau Ceti f. We are glad that representatives of Earth could find their way here. We have much to discuss. First, what are your intentions for this visit?"

"First, our intentions include establishing a peaceful relationship with Tau Ceti," said Erik. "We hope to conduct an exchange of information between us that will be of benefit to both races."

"We have been observing Earth for over 200 of your years," began Jarvait. "Your race appeared to be primitive to us. Warring amongst yourselves, nation against nation with senseless killing. We hoped that, as technology closed the distances that separated you, that you would abandon your territorial disputes and become one race as we have. Unfortunately, we see little progress in that regard.

"Our races have much in common, but we abhor violence. We see a tremendous amount of violence on Earth. In fact, it appears to be getting worse. Nuclear arms continue to threaten Earth's very existence. Greed and power seem to be the primary objectives of Earth's largest nation states. Efforts to enslave billions of your people are increasing in intensity.

"We suspect that one of your primary objectives is to gain knowledge of our wormhole technology. I will tell you now that Tau will not support or accommodate your race spreading violence and greed among the stars."

After a few moments, Erik responded. "I cannot deny that your concerns are valid. Human history is rife with bloodshed and death. And, honestly, the situation has not improved. Indeed, it has only worsened as our weaponry advanced, particularly in the past one hundred years. But I call to your attention that we have survived over forty centuries as an indigenous species. Our technology has taken us to the precipice of interstellar space travel. Many believe that, once achieved, space will be a unifying force for humankind."

"Perhaps, if you allow us, we can assist with efforts to unify Earth under a banner of peace," said Jarvait. "I will need to propose a plan to our government to do this. But we have done this for other races that were preparing to travel to the stars. Do you believe Earth would be receptive to our intervention in your… evolution?"

Silent for a few moments, Erik said, "Personally, I believe your offer of guidance to help Earth become an acceptable space-faring race is incredible. But convincing Earth's governments to embrace a transition to a global society would be formidable. Attempts like this in the past have failed. Would Tau support a delegation of Tau representatives coming to Earth to help introduce a plan? Actually, seeing another advanced race from space would be an excellent unifying force for Earth's people."

"What you suggest actually happened centuries ago to the Tau. After engaging another advanced race to aid Tau in overcoming division among its people," said Jarvait. "Tau overwhelmingly united. It is highly likely Tau would engage with you, as you suggest."

Later that evening, Erik lay down to rest his mind and recharge his synthetic body. Soon a familiar mist formed, and The Guardian materialized with another supernatural being. "Guardian, I was not expecting to see you here," said Erik.

"I bring another Guardian with me. He is known as Uhlan by Tau who know him, which translates to Guardian. We have listened to your conversations with Jarvait and unquestionably support what is developing. Know that together, we will assist in the unification of Earth."

Epilogue

Erik and crew remained on Tau Ceti f for several months as Jarvait introduced them to the Tau Council of Elders that oversaw the laws and cultures of the Tau people. The Council worked with local Tau governments to ensure that the accepted cultural norms were followed. The crew from Earth learned much about Tau history, including how they transitioned from a tribal, warlike existence to a peaceful, space-faring race. A plan being developed proposed a delegation of Tau Elders that would travel to Earth and serve as ambassadors The ambassadors would be introduced at the United Nations to present a brief history of the Tau, emphasizing their transition from a warlike race to one promoting peace and expansion beyond their solar system. Concepts presented to the UN would show that it was possible, and beneficial, for governments to exist peacefully with each other under a philosophy of mutual co-existence. The goal of the delegation would be to gain acceptance for Tau representatives to come to Earth and work with the UN Security Council nations to develop the basis and plans for peaceful coexistence. The Guardian and Uhlan, the guardian of Tau, would observe progress and initiate supernatural intervention to correct any disruptions to the developing timeline.

Begun in the 2010s by the World Economic Forum, efforts towards domination and enslavement of the masses continued. A global consortium of billionaire elites, bearing the name Future Earth, was formed. The cabal was intent on leveraging advanced AI technology to force complete adoption of digital passports, social credit scores for individuals, and ESG, environmental-social governance, for businesses. Just when the global elites were about to achieve their dystopian goals, the Tau delegation arrived at the United Nations. Future Earth then invested heavily in attacking the Tau proposal by saying it was a threat of conquest of Earth by the Tau. Use of the corporate media in promoting the lie was nearly universal. Future Earth immediately became a serious threat to the transition of Earth's governments to a peaceful, space-faring coalition.

Kristian Barnett returned to public life when he stated that Dr. Savannah Richards' cure for amyotrophic lateral sclerosis resulted in arresting the progress of the disease as well as restored his body to full functionality. Kristian continued to fight against the enslavement of humankind, leveraging his wealth and relationship with Senator Richards, who was elected President of the United States in 2052. Kristian and Ansley Barnett's daughter, Kristen Elaine, followed her mother into medicine with intentions of joining her mother's field of synthetics.

Aaron and Dr. Savannah Richards were married and were expecting their first child. News of the pregnancy sent Ksenia into a brief depression. Ksenia knew she could not bear children when she was injured and subsequently transitioned to a synthetic body. Ansley could not offer a means for Ksenia to become pregnant in her synthetic body. The only option open to Ksenia and Erik for children would be to enlist a surrogate.

The eternal battle between good and evil continues in Shepherds of Destiny III.

About the Author

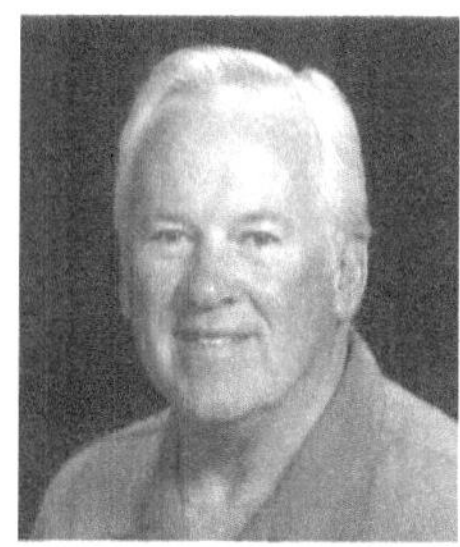

Kiel Barnekov is an information technology executive who has led innovative airline and airport technology projects for over thirty years. He was Director of Information Technology for Tampa International Airport and Manager of Information Technology at Orlando International Airport. He was also the Business Technology leader for Delta Air Lines Airport Customer Service Division during the 1990s. Well known in the airport industry, Mr. Barnekov has chaired the Airports Council International - North America Information Technology Committee. Mr. Barnekov as appeared on CNN and several local news stations to demonstrate airport technologies and airport processes. Shepherds of Destiny is Mr. Barnekov's first novel. He was born in 1951 in Washington D.C. His father was a federal government intelligence executive & captain in the U.S. Naval Reserve. His mother was a federal government employee at several agencies. His grandmother, Fleur Conkling, was a published author of children's books. Mr. Barnekov lives with his family in Ormond Beach, Florida.

Contact: Kiel.Barnekov@yahoo.com